NEONATAL AND PEDIATRIC CARDIOPULMONARY CARE

NEONATAL AND PEDIATRIC CARDIOPULMONARY CARE—A Self-Assessment

1200 Questions with Referenced Answers

THOMAS J. WILLIAMS, B.S., A.R.R.T.
Clinical Applications Specialist
Bourns, Inc.
Life Systems Division
Riverside, California 92506

YEAR BOOK MEDICAL PUBLISHERS, INC.
35 East Wacker Drive/Chicago

Library of Congress Catalog Card Number: 75-27702

International Standard Book Number: 0-8151-9302-5

To

MY WIFE
for her love, support and encouragement

MY FATHER
for teaching me the convictions which guide my life

MY MOTHER
for her kindness, patience and constant understanding

MY SON
for making everything I do worthwhile

PREFACE

This review book is intended for respiratory therapists, physicians, cardiopulmonary technologists, nurses and physical therapists interested in the ever-increasing realm of pediatric cardiopulmonary care. Its purpose is to challenge the clinician's mastery of several fundamental and advanced concepts which should be fully grasped to effectively care for infants and children. Thus, this text may be used as a review for registry and certification examinations as well as for self-evaluation. To accomplish this goal, the book has been designed to formulate both multiple choice and matching questions on a wide variety of topics inherent to cardiopulmonary care.

Because a diversity of opinion is often encountered in this type of endeavor, all the answers provided have been meticulously referenced. The reader should understand, however, that medical authorities often disagree among themselves. To this end it will not be surprising to encounter differing opinions on various answers. This is both expected and welcomed. When the clinician mentally challenges the author of a book, it fosters learning. This stimulates the pursuance of other texts and ultimately leads to a better, more informed individual. With greater over-all knowledge, the clinician is thus provided with a larger armamentarium of knowledge to incorporate in treating infants and children with cardiopulmonary disorders.

ACKNOWLEDGMENTS

In the preparation of this review book, special thanks must be extended to three of my colleagues who spent countless hours evaluating and constructively criticizing this manuscript. The valuable comments and helpful suggestions of Larry Fields, B.S., A.R.R.T.; Mary Garavaglia, B.S., A.R.R.T.; and Audrey Dennis, A.R.R.T., are warmly appreciated.

THOMAS J. WILLIAMS

TABLE OF CONTENTS

SECTION 1

Anatomy, Physiology and Terminology

For each of these questions select the *one* most appropriate answer.

1. The study of disorders of the newborn is called:
a. neonatology
b. obstetrics
c. pediatrics
d. perinatology
e. epidemiology *Ref. 1, p. 832*

2. The study of those events focusing on the child just before and after birth is the profession of:
a. perinatology
b. neonatology
c. pediatrics
d. obstetrics
e. gynecology *Ref. 2, p. vii*

3. The study and treatment of children in health and disease is called:
a. neonatology
b. obstetrics
c. pediatrics
d. gynecology
e. epidemiology *Ref. 1, p. 932*

4. The term gestation is most closely related to:
a. trimester
b. embryo
c. pregnancy
d. conception
e. birth *Ref. 1, p. 517*

5. An embryo is considered a fertilized ovum and remains so until organogenesis is completed. This occurs at:
a. 8 weeks
b. 10 weeks
c. 12 weeks
d. 14 weeks
e. 16 weeks *Ref. 3, p. 17*

6. An embryo becomes a fetus after:
a. 4 weeks
b. 6 weeks
c. 8 weeks
d. 10 weeks
e. 12 weeks *Ref. 3, p. 17*

7. The term neonate is synonymous with:
a. newborn
b. birth
c. infant
d. gestation
e. premature *Ref. 1, p. 832*

8. The neonatal period is:
a. the time just before birth
b. 2 weeks before birth and birth itself
c. the time succeeding birth and continuing through the first 2 weeks of life
d. the time succeeding birth and continuing through the first month of life
e. none of these *Ref. 1, p. 832*

9. The number of completed weeks which have elapsed between the first day of the last normal menstrual period and delivery of the fetus is called:
a. birth
b. gestational age
c. first trimester
d. neonatal period
e. none of these *Ref. 3, p. 16*

10. The first trimester is the period from the first day of the last normal menstrual period to:
a. 10 weeks
b. 13 weeks
c. 16 weeks
d. 18 weeks
e. 20 weeks *Ref. 3, p. 17*

11. The neonatal period is the interval from the time of birth up to:
a. 7 days
b. 14 days
c. 21 days
d. 28 days
e. 30 days *Ref. 3, p. 18*

12. The term fetus is most appropriately used:
a. after conception
b. after the first month of gestation
c. after the second month of gestation
d. during the 9-month pregnancy period
e. none of these *Ref. 3, p. 17*

13. The first anatomical evidence of fetal lung development occurs at:
a. 3.5 weeks
b. 6 weeks
c. 8 weeks
d. 12 weeks
e. 16 weeks *Ref. 4, p. 44*

14. An infant born before 38 weeks of gestation is called:
a. preterm
b. post-term
c. term
d. stillborn
e. postpartum *Ref. 3, p. 19*

15. An infant born in the 4-week period between 38 weeks' and 41 weeks' plus 6 days' gestation is called:

a. preterm
b. post-term
c. term
d. neonate
e. premature *Ref. 3, p. 19*

16. An infant is considered postmature if he is born after ______ weeks of gestation.

a. 36
b. 38
c. 40
d. 42
e. none of these *Ref. 2, p. 88*

17. Another name for childbirth is:

a. parturition
b. labor
c. delivery
d. all of these
e. a and c *Ref. 1, p. 236*

18. Childhood is the period of life:

a. immediately preceding birth
b. between birth and infancy
c. between infancy and puberty
d. following puberty
e. preceding birth and up to puberty

Ref. 1, p. 236

19. A stillborn infant:

a. is not a fetus
b. has a heartbeat but no respirations
c. has respirations but no heartbeat
d. shows no evidence of life
e. shows only minimal evidence of life

Ref. 3, p. 18

20. The process by which a live-born infant or a stillborn infant is expelled or extracted from the mother is called:

a. birth

b. death
c. preterm
d. abortion
e. gestation *Ref. 3, p. 17*

21. Perinatal death is an all-inclusive term referring to:
a. stillborn deaths
b. neonatal deaths
c. all premature infant deaths
d. all infant deaths
e. both stillborn infants and neonatal deaths
Ref. 3, p. 23

22. A low birth weight infant is one who weighs less than ______ gm at birth.
a. 2500
b. 3000
c. 3500
d. 4000
e. 4500 *Ref. 5, p. 421*

23. The organ of metabolic interchange between the fetus and mother is the:
a. foramen ovale
b. amniotic fluid
c. umbilical cord
d. placenta
e. none of these *Ref. 2, p. 1*

24. The term premature most accurately describes:
a. infants born before the 37th week of gestation
b. infants less than 2500 gm
c. infants of low birth weight
d. all of these
e. a and c *Ref. 2, p. 86*

25. An infant who weighs 2251 gm is ______ lb.
a. 3 lb
b. 4 lb
c. 5 lb
d. 8 lb
e. 9 lb *Ref. 6, p. 209*

26. The length of the average newborn is:
a. 12 in.
b. 14 in.
c. 16 in.
d. 20 in.
e. 25 in. *Ref. 7, p. 74*

27. The weight of the average newborn is:
a. 2–4 lb
b. 4–6 lb
c. 6–8 lb
d. 8–10 lb
e. over 10 lb *Ref. 7, p. 74*

28. The skin at birth is ordinarily covered with:
a. ligamentum nuchae
b. pseudostratified ciliated columnar epithelium
c. vernix caseosa
d. bile
e. meconium *Ref. 8, p. 190*

29. The purpose of silver nitrate administration to the eyes of newborn infants is:
a. irrigation of the retina
b. prevention of retrolental fibroplasia
c. prophylaxis against gonorrheal infection
d. visualization of the blink reflex
e. reduction of edema *Ref. 2, p. 51*

30. At birth the percent of total body weight which is water is:
a. 50%
b. 60%
c. 70%
d. 80%
e. 90% *Ref. 9, p. 304*

31. A 1½-kg baby would weigh:
a. 0.92 lb
b. 1.4 lb
c. 2.2 lb

d. 3.3 lb
e. 4.4 lb *Ref. 1, p. 669*

32. The external openings of the nose are called:
a. septum
b. turbinates
c. nares
d. vomer
e. vestibule *Ref. 10, p. 921*

33. The external openings of the nose are separated from each other by the:
a. nostrils
b. nasal septum
c. nares
d. turbinates
e. vomer *Ref. 10, p. 921*

34. The function of the nose is to:
a. warm the inspired air
b. moisten the inspired air
c. filter the inspired air
d. all of these
e. a and b *Ref. 11, p. 465*

35. Turbinates are found in the:
a. nose
b. larynx
c. pharynx
d. trachea
e. bronchi *Ref. 10, p. 924*

36. Another name for turbinate is:
a. septum
b. atrium
c. arch
d. conchae
e. sinus *Ref. 10, p. 924*

37. Cilia serve to:

a. filter the inspired air
b. warm the exhaled air
c. propel secretions toward the oropharynx
d. all of these
e. a and c *Ref. 12, p. 36*

38. The cilia constantly propel the mucous blanket toward the:

a. nares
b. nose
c. turbinates
d. pharynx
e. none of these *Ref. 11, p. 465*

39. Which of the following is divisible into nasal, oral and laryngeal regions?

a. nose
b. pharynx
c. larynx
d. trachea
e. bronchi *Ref. 10, p. 937*

40. At what level is the neonate's larynx at birth?

a. first cervical vertebra
b. fourth cervical vertebra
c. fifth cervical vertebra
d. first thoracic vertebra
e. second thoracic vertebra *Ref. 4, p. 143*

41. At birth the cricoid cartilage is at the level of the:

a. first cervical vertebra
b. second cervical vertebra
c. third cervical vertebra
d. fourth cervical vertebra
e. fifth cervical vertebra *Ref. 4, p. 144*

42. The largest cartilage present in the larynx is the:

a. thyroid
b. cricoid
c. arytenoid

d. epiglottic
e. none of these *Ref. 10, p. 945*

43. Which of the following cartilages in the larynx are paired?
a. arytenoid
b. thyroid
c. cricoid
d. epiglottic
e. a and c *Ref. 13, p. 518*

44. In the neonate the distance from the larynx to the carina is:
a. 1 in.
b. 4.0 cm
c. 2.54 cm
d. 5.7 cm
e. 3.5 cm *Ref. 14, p. 994*

45. The glottis is protected by a lip of fibrocartilage called the:
a. thyroid cartilage
b. cricoid cartilage
c. arytenoid cartilage
d. epiglottis
e. cuneiform cartilage *Ref. 13, p. 519*

46. The opening between the vocal cords is called the:
a. glottis
b. epiglottis
c. oropharynx
d. turbinates
e. stoma *Ref. 13, p. 519*

47. The area of the trachea that separates the openings of the two principal bronchi is termed the:
a. hilum
b. T_4
c. carina
d. lingula
e. T_7 *Ref. 10, p. 514*

48. The diameter of the infant trachea is:
a. 1.0–2.0 cm
b. 2.0–3.0 cm
c. 3.5–4.0 cm
d. 4.0–5.0 cm
e. 5.0–5.5 cm *Ref. 4, p. 143*

49. The length of the infant trachea is:
a. 1–2 cm
b. 2–4 cm
c. 5 cm
d. 5–6 cm
e. 6–8 cm *Ref. 4, p. 149*

50. The cartilaginous rings in the trachea are:
a. complete
b. C-shaped
c. concentric
d. rectangular
e. cylindrical *Ref. 13, p. 522*

51. The trachea divides into the left and right main stem bronchi at the:
a. esophagus
b. larynx
c. bifurcation
d. carina
e. c and d *Ref. 10, p. 514*

52. The type of cartilage found in the trachea is:
a. hyaline
b. fibrous
c. elastic
d. costal
e. articular *Ref. 13, p. 522*

53. In all children over the age of 3 years, the subcarinal angle between the two main bronchi is:
a. 45 degrees
b. 50 degrees
c. 56 degrees
d. 62 degrees
e. 70 degrees *Ref. 15, p. 341*

54. In all children over the age of 3 years, the right principal bronchus leaves the trachea at an angle of:

a. 25 degrees
b. 30 degrees
c. 35 degrees
d. 40 degrees
e. 45 degrees *Ref. 10, p. 514*

55. In all children over the age of 3 years, the left principal bronchus leaves the trachea at an angle of:

a. 30 degrees
b. 37 degrees
c. 40 degrees
d. 45 degrees
e. 50 degrees *Ref. 15, p. 341*

56. The right principal bronchus gives off its first branch close to the:

a. lingula
b. middle lobe
c. hilum
d. inferior lobe
e. posterior basal segment *Ref. 10, p. 519*

57. In all children under the age of 3 years, the right and left main stem bronchi diverge from the trachea at:

a. 25 degrees left, 45 degrees right
b. 25 degrees right, 45 degrees left
c. 55 degrees right, 55 degrees left
d. 35 degrees left, 50 degrees right
e. 35 degrees right, 50 degrees left

Ref. 16, p. 466

58. Which of the following is a branch off the right main stem bronchus?

a. superior lobe bronchus
b middle lobe bronchus
c. inferior lobe bronchus
d. eparterial bronchus
e. all of these *Ref. 15, p. 341*

59. How many divisions of the bronchial tree are present at birth?

a. 12
b. 14
c. 17
d. 20
e. 23 *Ref. 17, p. 483*

60. The lungs are anatomically divided into areas called lobes. How many lobes are there in both lungs?

a. 2
b. 3
c. 5
d. 7
e. 9 *Ref. 10, p. 509*

61. The right lung has how many lobes?

a. 2
b. 3
c. 4
d. 5
e. 6 *Ref. 10, p. 509*

62. The left lung has how many lobes?

a. 2
b. 3
c. 5
d. 6
e. 7 *Ref. 10, p. 509*

63. What are the divisions between the lobes called?

a. apex
b. base
c. hilum
d. fissure
e. lingula *Ref. 10, p. 509*

64. A part of a lobe of a lung that is supplied by a bronchus is called a:

a. hilum
b. bronchopulmonary segment
c. lingula

d. fissure
e. division *Ref. 10, p. 518*

65. The right lung has:
a. 3 bronchopulmonary segments
b. 4 bronchopulmonary segments
c. 6 bronchopulmonary segments
d. 8 bronchopulmonary segments
e. 10 bronchopulmonary segments *Ref. 18, p. 10*

66. The left lung has:
a. 3 bronchopulmonary segments
b. 4 bronchopulmonary segments
c. 6 bronchopulmonary segments
d. 8 bronchopulmonary segments
e. 10 bronchopulmonary segments *Ref. 18, p. 10*

67. Which of these statements concerning the lungs is false?
a. the right lung is larger, shorter and wider than the left lung
b. the lung is highly elastic
c. the left lung has a greater volume than the right lung
d. the normal human lung is pink
e. the surface of the lung is covered by visceral pleura
Ref. 15, p. 343

68. In the human, the lung carries out which of the following physiologic functions?
a. gas exchange
b. filtering toxic substances
c. a reservoir of blood
d. metabolism
e. all of these *Ref. 19, p. 1*

69. The middle lobe of the right lung corresponds to what anatomical portion of the left lung?
a. hilum
b. fissure
c. lingula
d. upper lobe
e. lower segment *Ref. 15, p. 345*

70. The homologue of the lingula of the left lung is the:
a. superior lobe of the right lung
b. middle lobe of the right lung
c. inferior lobe of the right lung
d. oblique fissure
e. horizontal fissure *Ref. 15, p. 345*

71. Each lung is connected to the heart and trachea by:
a. bronchial arteries and veins
b. the pulmonary artery and vein
c. plexuses of nerves
d. lymphatics and lymph nodes
e. all of these *Ref. 13. p. 524*

72. Blood supply to the lungs originates from the:
a. pulmonary artery
b. bronchial artery
c. subclavian artery
d. carotid artery
e. a and b *Ref. 13, p. 525*

73. The area of the lung in which innervating structures enter and exit the lung is called the:
a. apex
b. base
c. hilum
d. notch
e. fissure *Ref. 10, p. 508*

74. The terminal bronchiole gives rise to the:
a. respiratory bronchiole
b. alveolar duct
c. alveolar sac
d. alveoli
e. alveolar duct and alveolar sac simultaneously *Ref. 15, p. 346*

75. Each respiratory bronchiole gives rise to how many alveolar ducts?
a. 2
b. 2–4
c. 1–8

d. 2–11
e. 1–20 *Ref. 15, p. 346*

76. The shape of the alveoli is:
a. polyhedral
b. cuboidal
c. sphenoidal
d. round
e. triangular *Ref. 15, p. 346*

77. The functional respiratory unit does not include:
a. terminal bronchiole
b. respiratory bronchiole
c. alveolar duct
d. atria
e. alveoli *Ref. 11, p. 476*

78. Which of the following is not a conducting airway?
a. alveoli
b. respiratory bronchiole
c. terminal bronchiole
d. bronchus
e. trachea *Ref. 19, p. 2*

79. Which blood vessel supplies the respiratory bronchioles, alveolar ducts and alveoli?
a. capillaries
b. bronchial artery
c. pulmonary artery
d. innominate artery
e. carotid artery *Ref. 12, p. 29*

80. The average newborn infant has how much anatomical deadspace?
a. 10.0 ml
b. 8.6 ml
c. 4.4 ml
d. 3.0 ml
e. 7.0 ml *Ref. 20, p. 158*

81. Particles which deposit in the alveoli are removed by:
a. cilia
b. red blood cells
c. macrophages
d. platelets
e. none of these *Ref. 19, p. 12*

82. A chemical substance in the alveoli which varies surface tension as alveolar volume changes is:
a. acetylcholine
b. norepinephrine
c. surfactant
d. carbonic anhydrase
e. DNA *Ref. 12, p. 58*

83. Which of the following does not refer to pulmonary surfactant?
a. dipalmityl lecithin
b. phospholipid
c. derived from type II alveolar cells
d. increases surface tension
e. a deficiency causes respiratory distress syndrome *Ref. 4, p. 46*

84. Lecithin:
a. does not increase surface tension
b. is part of the L/S ratio
c. is synthesized by two pathways
d. is analyzed following amniocentesis
e. all of these *Ref. 21, p. 223*

85. The normal L/S ratio at term is at least:
a. 1.5
b. 1.7
c. 1.9
d. 2.1
e. 2.4 *Ref. 22, p. 212*

86. A deficiency of pulmonary surfactant:
a. increases compliance
b. decreases compliance
c. decreases airway resistance

d. increases Pa_{O_2}
e. causes even distribution of inspired gas

Ref. 12, p. 59

87. Another name for the sternum is the:
a. manubrium
b. body
c. xiphoid process
d. breastbone
e. sternal notch *Ref. 10, p. 497*

88. The composition of the sternum does not include the:
a. manubrium
b. body
c. gladiolus
d. tubercle
e. xiphoid process *Ref. 13, p. 116*

89. The lowest anatomical division of the sternum is called the:
a. manubrium
b. body
c. xiphoid process
d. breastbone
e. sternal notch *Ref. 10, p. 497*

90. Another name for the xiphoid process is the:
a. ensiform
b. gladiolus
c. tubercle
d. costae
e. trochanter *Ref. 13, p. 116*

91. Which of these statements concerning the ribs is false?
a. there are 12 pairs of ribs
b. the first 7 ribs are called true ribs
c. the lower 5 ribs are called floating ribs
d. the first 7 ribs are attached to the sternum through costal cartilage
e. the terms floating ribs and false ribs are not the same *Ref. 10, p. 497*

92. The area between the two pleural sacs is the:

a. heart
b. trachea
c. esophagus
d. mediastinum
e. sternum *Ref. 10, p. 504*

93. The thoracic mediastinum is composed of all of the following except the:

a. superior mediastinum
b. middle mediastinum
c. inferior mediastinum
d. posterior mediastinum
e. anterior mediastinum *Ref. 15, p. 315*

94. A structure not found in the mediastinum is the:

a. trachea
b. heart
c. lungs
d. esophagus
e. superior vena cava *Ref. 10, p. 505*

95. Which of these muscles plays no active part in any type of inspiration?

a. diaphragm
b. external intercostals
c. internal intercostals
d. sternocleidomastoid
e. pectoralis minor *Ref. 13, p. 530*

96. Which of these statements concerning lung development is false?

a. at 28 days two primary branches appear which will become major bronchi
b. at 10 weeks cartilage deposition begins
c. at 16 weeks formation of the bronchi is nearly complete
d. by the 12th week the lobes of the lung may be demarcated
e. alveolar formation stops before term

Ref. 23, pp. 3–4

97. Which of the following statements is false concerning infants?

a. the larynx is more cephalad
b. the epiglottis is longer and stiffer than in an adult
c. the vocal cords are the narrowest point of the larynx
d. the infant has a proportionately large tongue at birth
e. the diameter of the trachea is 3.5–4.0 mm

Ref. 4, p. 144

98. Regarding children, which of the following statements is false?

a. the nasal passages are narrow
b. the tongue is relatively large
c. the epiglottis is shorter than in an adult
d. the epiglottis is V-shaped
e. the vocal cords are concave *Ref. 24, p. 127*

99. Which of the following statements is false?

a. neonates are obligatory mouth breathers
b. thoracic retraction is a sign of labored breathing in the infant
c. the average respiratory rate in infants is 40 breaths per minute
d. the thorax of the infant is flexible
e. an expiratory grunt creates back pressure on the airway *Ref. 4, p. 2*

100. Which of the following statements is *not* false?

a. the trachea narrows on inspiration
b. the trachea dilates on expiration
c. the trachea collapses on inspiration
d. the trachea narrows on expiration
e. the trachea never changes shape during the normal respiratory cycle *Ref. 24, p. 128*

101. The structural differences of the upper airways in the infant compared with those of the adult are:

a. the nasal passages are narrow
b. the tongue is proportionally large
c. the glottis is higher
d. the cricoid ring is small
e. all of these *Ref. 25, p. 97*

102. The medulla contains:
a. inspiratory and expiratory centers
b. inspiratory center only
c. expiratory center only
d. carotid bodies
e. all of the cranial nerves *Ref. 4, p. 5*

103. Prolonged stimulation of the apneustic center causes:
a. apnea
b. hyperpnea
c. prolonged inspiration
d. prolonged expiration
e. tachycardia *Ref. 26, p. 68*

104. Which of the following terms does not pertain to the heart?
a. pericardium
b. myocardium
c. epicardium
d. duocardium
e. endocardium *Ref. 13, p. 383*

105. The pericardium is the:
a. internal layer of the heart
b. middle layer of the heart
c. serous membrane covering the heart
d. area of the heart which covers the valves
e. none of these *Ref. 13, pp. 383, 384*

106. The middle layer of the heart is the:
a. pericardium
b. epicardium
c. duocardium
d. myocardium
e. endocardium *Ref. 13, p. 384*

107. The internal layer of the heart is the:
a. pericardium
b. epicardium
c. duocardium
d. myocardium
e. endocardium *Ref. 13, p. 384*

108. The valve located between the right atrium and right ventricle is the:
a. tricuspid
b. bicuspid
c. mitral
d. pulmonary
e. aortic *Ref. 13, p. 388*

109. The valve located between the left atrium and left ventricle is the:
a. tricuspid
b. mitral
c. aortic
d. pulmonary
e. semilunar *Ref. 13, p. 388*

110. Another name for the pulmonary and aortic valves is:
a. tricuspid valves
b. bicuspid valves
c. semilunar valves
d. mitral valves
e. coronary valves *Ref. 13, p. 389*

111. The number of cusps or flaps present in the composition of the tricuspid valve is:
a. 1
b. 2
c. 3
d. 4
e. 5 *Ref. 13, p. 388*

112. The number of cusps or flaps present in the composition of the mitral valve is:
a. 1
b. 2
c. 3
d. 4
e. 5 *Ref. 13, p. 388*

113. The number of cusps or flaps present in the composition of the semilunar valves is:
a. 1
b. 2
c. 3
d. 4
e. 5 *Ref. 13, p. 389*

114. In a child, blood from the superior and inferior venae cavae enters the heart at the:
a. right atrium
b. left atrium
c. right ventricle
d. left ventricle
e. aorta *Ref. 13, p. 442*

115. In a child, blood from the right ventricle goes to the:
a. lungs
b. aorta
c. pulmonary artery
d. left atrium
e. body *Ref. 13, p. 443*

116. In a child, blood from the lungs enters the left atrium via the:
a. pulmonary artery
b. pulmonary veins
c. aorta
d. innominate artery
e. all of these *Ref. 13, p. 442*

117. The total number of pulmonary veins which emerge from the lung is:
a. 1
b. 2
c. 3
d. 4
e. 5 *Ref. 13, p. 442*

118. At birth, or shortly thereafter, there is closure of which of the following?
a. ductus arteriosus

b. ductus venosus
c. foramen ovale
d. all of these
e. a and c *Ref. 27, p. 19*

119. Closure of the foramen ovale is very likely functionally complete within the first:
a. few minutes
b. day
c. 2–3 days
d. week
e. month *Ref. 27, p. 19*

120. Closure of the ductus arteriosus probably occurs during the first:
a. few minutes
b. 8 hours
c. day
d. 2–3 days
e. week *Ref. 27, p. 19*

121. When the umbilical cord is clamped and cut at birth there should be present:
a. 1 artery and 1 vein
b. 2 arteries
c. 2 veins
d. 2 arteries and 1 vein
e. 1 artery and 2 veins *Ref. 2, p. 51*

122. Hemoglobin may be described as:
a. the oxygen-carrying component of the blood
b. having greater affinity for carbon monoxide than for oxygen
c. a coloring component of whole blood
d. all of these
e. a and b *Ref. 28, pp. 33–35*

123. The hemoglobin of the fetus is predominantly:
a. hemoglobin A
b. hemoglobin F
c. hemoglobin S
d. hemoglobin H
e. none of these *Ref. 27, p. 19*

124. In a mature newborn infant the amount of adult hemoglobin (hemoglobin A) present is approximately:

a. 20%
b. 30%
c. 40%
d. 50%
e. 60% *Ref. 27, p. 19*

125. In the normal physiological state, fetal hemoglobin is replaced by adult hemoglobin at _____ after parturition.

a. 1 week
b. 1 month
c. 6 months
d. 1 year
e. 2 years *Ref. 12, p. 77*

126. The hemoglobin level of the newborn infant averages:

a. 8–10 gm
b. 10–12 gm
c. 13–15 gm
d. 15–17 gm
e. 17–19 gm *Ref. 27, p. 22*

127. Each 100 ml of blood with an oxygen tension of 100 mm Hg contains _____ of dissolved oxygen.

a. 0.03 ml
b. 0.003 ml
c. 0.3 ml
d. 20.0 ml
e. 80–100 ml *Ref. 28, p. 36*

128. Each 15 gm % of Hb will combine with _____ ml of oxygen.

a. 19.0
b. 19.6
c. 20.4
d. 0.3
e. 0.003 *Ref. 28, p. 36*

129. **One gram of hemoglobin can combine with approximately 1.34 ml oxygen. Multiplying this factor times 15 gm of hemoglobin per 100 ml plasma, one can arrive at the:**
a. amount of oxygen in solution
b. oxygen combined with hemoglobin
c. oxygen-carrying capacity of hemoglobin
d. PO_2
e. Pa_{O_2} *Ref. 28, p. 36*

130. **The amount of oxygen associated with a given amount of hemoglobin compared with the amount which would be present if the hemoglobin were fully saturated is:**
a. oxygen content
b. oxygen tension
c. oxygen saturation
d. oxygen-carrying capacity
e. oxygen affinity *Ref. 29, p. 447*

131. **The minimum amount of reduced (i.e., unoxygenated) hemoglobin required to produce cyanosis is:**
a. 1 gm
b. 4 gm
c. 5 gm
d. 8 gm
e. 10 gm *Ref. 28, p. 77*

132. **Cyanosis of the hands and feet is called:**
a. biocyanosis
b. acrocyanosis
c. trocyanosis
d. pallor
e. none of these *Ref. 30, p. 199*

133. **Cyanotic infants are susceptible to:**
a. hypothermia
b. hypotension
c. hypoglycemia
d. hypocalcemia
e. all of these *Ref. 31, p. 878*

134. In an infant, acrocyanosis usually disappears:
a. when the infant is transfused
b. after bringing the temperature to normal
c. when packed cells are given
d. following oxygen administration
e. when oxygen and blood are administered
Ref. 31, p. 878

135. Cyanosis is best treated by:
a. replacement of R.B.C.s
b. increasing FI_{O_2}
c. administration of plasma
d. transfusing A.C.D.-treated blood
e. all of these *Ref. 32, p. 155*

136. Cyanosis and hypoxemia may result from:
a. alveolar hypoventilation
b. a defect in gas diffusion
c. right-to-left shunting of blood
d. all of these
e. a and b *Ref. 29, p. 453*

137. Often an infant seems to show evidence of cyanosis because of:
a. the color of the wall paint
b. the type of lighting in the nursery
c. the infant's being hypothermic
d. the infant's being polycythemic
e. all of these *Ref. 33, p. 139*

138. The degree of visible cyanosis in a newborn does not depend on the:
a. hematocrit
b. pH
c. Pa_{CO_2}
d. peripheral circulation
e. arterial oxygen saturation *Ref. 33, p. 139*

139. In the neonate, cyanosis is first observed at oxygen tensions between:
a. 22–32 mm Hg
b. 32–42 mm Hg

c. 42–52 mm Hg
d. 52–62 mm Hg
e. 62–72 mm Hg *Ref. 25, p. 43*

140. In a newborn infant, pallor of the skin may indicate:
a. narcosis
b. shock
c. massive blood loss
d. all of these
e. a and c *Ref. 30, p. 201*

141. The percent of red blood cells in whole blood refers to:
a. hemoglobin
b. hypoxemia
c. hematocrit
d. oxygen content
e. hemolysis *Ref. 11, p. 204*

142. The enzyme carbonic anhydrase is found in red blood cells and:
a. brain cells
b. liver cells
c. kidney glomerular cells
d. spleen cells
e. kidney tubular cells *Ref. 28, p. 50*

143. The normal blood volume in an infant is:
a. 20 ml/kg of body weight
b. 40 ml/kg of body weight
c. 60 ml/kg of body weight
d. 80 ml/kg of body weight
e. 100 ml/kg of body weight *Ref. 33, p. 143*

144. The blood volume of the newborn is about _____ percent of his body weight.
a. 10–12
b. 18–20
c. 20–25
d. 25–30
e. 30–35 *Ref. 7, p. 78*

145. The oxygen dissociation curve of fetal blood is _____ as compared with adult hemoglobin.

a. shifted to the left
b. shifted to the right
c. not shifted
d. normally elevated
e. none of these *Ref. 25, p. 43*

146. The sum of the oxygen in combination with the hemoglobin plus that dissolved in plasma is the:

a. P_{50}
b. oxygen affinity
c. oxygen content
d. oxygen tension
e. Pa_{O_2} *Ref. 28, p. 35*

147. In order to correctly and effectively use the oxyhemoglobin dissociation curve, which of the following should be used in addition to the patient's PO_2?

a. body temperature
b. pH
c. PCO_2
d. all of these
e. a and b *Ref. 4, p. 27*

148. Which of the following does not shift the oxyhemoglobin dissociation curve to the right?

a. hyperthermia
b. acidosis
c. fetal hemoglobin
d. a and b
e. a and c *Ref. 29, p. 448*

149. On the fetal hemoglobin dissociation curve, cyanosis is first observed at an arterial oxygen saturation of:

a. 50%–60%
b. 60%–70%
c. 75%–85%
d. 80%–90%
e. 85%–95% *Ref. 33, p. 108*

150. On the fetal hemoglobin dissociation curve, cyanosis is first observed at a Pa_{O_2} level of:

a. 22–32 mm Hg
b. 32–42 mm Hg
c. 42–52 mm Hg
d. 52–62 mm Hg
e. 62–72 mm Hg *Ref. 33, p. 108*

151. An increase in oxygen affinity is indicative of which of the following?

a. left-sided shift in oxyhemoglobin dissociation curve
b. an increased affinity of oxygen to hemoglobin
c. a decreased affinity of oxygen to hemoglobin
d. right-sided shift in oxyhemoglobin dissociation curve
e. a and b *Ref. 28, p. 39*

152. At any Pa_{O_2} below 100 mm Hg:

a. fetal blood binds more oxygen
b. fetal blood binds no oxygen
c. fetal blood binds less oxygen
d. fetal blood is acidotic
e. fetal blood is alkalotic *Ref. 25, p. 43*

153. The partial pressure of oxygen at which hemoglobin is 50% saturated is the:

a. L/S ratio
b. P_{50}
c. hematocrit
d. % saturation
e. O_2 content *Ref. 34, p. 15*

154. What is P_{50}?

a. a PO_2 of 50 mm Hg
b. an isotope of oxygen
c. the value of PO_2 when hemoglobin is 50% saturated
d. a substance in the red blood cell
e. the isopleth of oxygen *Ref. 4, p. 28*

155. Determination of P_{50} is used to detect:
a. airway resistance
b. alveolar capillary block
c. shifts by the oxyhemoglobin dissociation curve
d. the ratio of red blood cells to hemoglobin
e. hypoxic hypoxia *Ref. 4, p. 28*

156. Which of the following factors causes a decrease in P_{50}?
a. increased vascular salts
b. methemoglobin
c. organic phosphates
d. increased temperature
e. decreased pH *Ref. 19, p. 76*

157. Blood stored in a blood bank for 5 days:
a. has a PO_2 of 50–75
b. has a decrease in 2,3-DPG
c. has an increase in PCO_2 to 90 mm Hg
d. will cause the patient to hypoventilate
e. none of these *Ref. 28, p. 99*

158. When blood is stored under standard conditions for more than several days the 2,3-DPG level:
a. increases
b. increases first, then gradually decreases
c. decreases
d. remains the same
e. decreases and subsequently increases P_{50}
Ref. 28, p. 99

159. Infants who receive fresh acid-citrate-dextrose (A.C.D.) blood in exchange tranfusions usually do better than those who receive stored blood; this is probably due to the:
a. increased number of red blood cells
b. increased amount of hemoglobin
c. higher 2,3-DPG content
d. lower 2,3-DPG content
e. increase of carbonic anhydrase *Ref. 4, p. 29*

160. Which statement is false concerning oxygen transport in a term infant?

a. P_{50} increases with age
b. the quantity of fetal hemoglobin decreases with age
c. the quantity of adult hemoglobin increases with age
d. P_{50} stays the same
e. the oxyhemoglobin curve is shifted to the left *Ref. 29, p. 450*

161. A child with severe anemia has hypoxia for which of the following reasons:

a. the blood has a reduced oxygen-carrying capacity
b. the hemoglobin is abnormal
c. the rate of blood flow is not fast enough
d. there is a huge shunt created
e. the 2,3-DPG level is unfavorably altered

Ref. 11, p. 105

162. The measurement of the arterial oxygen tension reflects the:

a. Pa_{O_2}
b. presence of hypoxemia
c. absence of hypoxemia
d. all of these
e. a and b *Ref. 28, p. 33*

163. An increased alveolar-to-arterial oxygen tension gradient indicates:

a. left-to-right shunt
b. right-to-left shunt
c. surfactant deficiency
d. none of these
e. all of these *Ref. 35, p. 232*

164. Oxygen and carbon dioxide move between air and blood by:

a. diffusion
b. osmosis
c. perfusion
d. Dalton's law
e. Poiseuille's law *Ref. 19, p. 1*

165. The largest fraction of CO_2 is carried as ______ in the blood.
a. dissolved CO_2
b. carbamino compound
c. H_2CO_3
d. carbaminohemoglobin
e. bicarbonate *Ref. 4, p. 31*

166. There is normally ______ mEq/L of dissolved CO_2 in the blood.
a. 1.2
b. 2.1
c. 6.0
d. 24.0
e. 28.0 *Ref. 26, p. 117*

167. Dissolved CO_2 in vol % = ______ × P_{CO_2}.
a. 0.0003
b. 0.003
c. 0.03
d. 0.3
e. 3.0 *Ref. 26, p. 116*

168. Total CO_2 is a combination of:
a. P_{CO_2} and dissolved CO_2
b. P_{CO_2} and combined CO_2
c. dissolved CO_2 and combined CO_2
d. Pa_{CO_2} and Pe_{CO_2}
e. none of these *Ref. 26, p. 115*

169. The normal alveolar-to-arterial oxygen tension gradient in early infancy with the infant breathing room air is:
a. zero
b. 20 mm Hg
c. 30 mm Hg
d. 40 mm Hg
e. 104 mm Hg *Ref. 35, p. 232*

170. The detection of hypoxemia is ordinarily based upon:
a. cyanosis
b. laboratory estimation of Pa_{O_2}
c. hemoglobin saturation

d. oxyhemoglobin saturation
e. all of these *Ref. 36, p. 4*

171. $P_B = P_{N_2} + P_{O_2} + P_{CO_2} + P_{H_2O}$ is whose law?
a. Boyle's law
b. Charles' law
c. Dalton's law
d. Henry's law
e. Graham's law *Ref. 12, p. 19*

172. The partial pressure of a gas is found by multiplying its:
a. concentration by the total barometric pressure
b. total pressure minus water vapor by the concentration
c. water-vapor tension by the concentration
d. concentration by the total pressure and then subtracting the water-vapor tension
e. total pressure by the water-vapor tension
Ref. 19, p. 1

173. The normal ambient partial pressures in the lung (at the alveolar level) are approximately:
a. P_{N_2} 400, P_{CO_2} 40, P_{O_2} 100
b. P_{N_2} 560, P_{CO_2} 47, P_{O_2} 100
c. P_{N_2} 600, P_{CO_2} 47, P_{O_2} 80
d. P_{N_2} 600, P_{CO_2} 40, P_{O_2} 120
e. none of these *Ref. 11, p. 474*

174. Volume = pressure × solubility coefficient is whose law?
a. Henry's law
b. Gay-Lussac's law
c. Poiseuille's law
d. Dalton's law
e. Hooke's law *Ref. 11, p. 472*

175. The formula $\dot{V} = \frac{P \cdot r^4}{8 \cdot L \cdot N}$ is known as:
a. Boyle's law
b. Hooke's law
c. Poiseuille's law
d. Reynolds' law
e. the Bohr equation *Ref. 19, p. 103*

176. Which of the following is a synonym for compliance?

a. resistance
b. distensibility
c. elasticity
d. sensitivity
e. volume *Ref. 12, p. 54*

177. Volume change per unit pressure change describes:

a. resistance
b. compliance
c. flow
d. cardiac output
e. shunt *Ref. 19, p. 155*

178. $\dot{V}_A$ stands for:

a. tidal volume
b. minute volume
c. alveolar ventilation
d. volume ventilation
e. ventilation per unit pressure *Ref. 26, p. 57*

179. The average lung ventilation-perfusion ratio is:

a. 1:200
b. 20:1
c. 4:5
d. 0.05
e. 5:4 *Ref. 26, p. 172*

180. For a normal resting infant the $\dot{V}_A/\dot{Q}_C$ is:

a. 0.45
b. 0.55
c. 0.65
d. 0.80
e. 0.90 *Ref. 35, p. 231*

181. Neither ventilated nor perfused describes:

a. shunt
b. silent unit
c. deadspace
d. all of these
e. none of these *Ref. 28, p. 69*

182. Perfused but not ventilated describes:
a. shunt
b. deadspace
c. foramen ovale
d. pores of Kohn
e. none of these *Ref. 37, p. 12*

183. Ventilated but not perfused describes:
a. alveolar deadspace
b. shunt
c. alveolar air
d. pores of Kohn
e. the alveolocapillary membrane

Ref. 11, p. 464

184. Which formula best represents alveolar ventilation?
a. $(V_A - V_D) = D_S$
b. $(V_T - V_D) \times F = \dot{V}_A$
c. $V_1/T_1 = V_2/T_2$
d. $V = P/T$
e. $(V_D - V_T) \times F = V_A$ *Ref. 11, p. 464*

185. The diffusion of gases through the respiratory membrane is dependent on:
a. the thickness of the membrane
b. the surface area of the membrane
c. the diffusion coefficient of the gas
d. the pressure difference between the two sides of the membrane
e. all of these *Ref. 11, p. 478*

186. Mouth pressure − alveolar pressure ÷ flow equals:
a. compliance
b. airway resistance
c. volume
d. output
e. solubility *Ref. 4, p. 19*

187. Another name for physiological deadspace is:

a. anatomical deadspace
b. alveolar deadspace
c. mechanical deadspace
d. a and b
e. b and c *Ref. 26, p. 56*

188. In a newborn infant a rare occurrence is:

a. a sneeze
b. a cry
c. an increased temperature
d. a cough
e. an increased respiratory rate *Ref. 39, p. 312*

189. The partial pressure of water in the lungs of a child at 5000 ft (P_B = 632.5 mm Hg) and ambient temperature of 37 C is equal to:

a. 20 mm Hg
b. 47 mm Hg
c. 100 mm Hg
d. 104 mm Hg
e. 159 mm Hg *Ref. 12, p. 20*

In column A are listed the most frequently used symbols of pulmonary physiology. In column B are listed the definitions of these symbols. Match column A with column B.

Column A	Column B
190. ______ $\dot{V}$	a. diffusing capacity
191. ______ $\bar{V}$	b. respiratory exchange ratio
192. ______ P	c. mean gas pressure
193. ______ $\bar{P}$	d. gas volume
194. ______ F	e. gas volume per unit time
195. ______ D	f. gas pressure
196. ______ R	g. fractional concentration
197. ______ I	h. deadspace gas
198. ______ E	i. barometric
199. ______ A	j. inspired gas
200. ______ T	k. alveolar gas
201. ______ D	l. expired gas
202. ______ B	m. tidal gas
203. ______ STPD	

204. ______ BTPS
205. ______ ATPS

n. ambient temperature and pressure saturated with water vapor
o. 0 C, 760 mm Hg dry
p. body temperature and pressure saturated with water vapor

Ref. 38, p. 330

In column A are listed some common examples frequently encountered in pulmonary physiology for gases. In column B are listed the definitions of these examples. Match column A with column B.

Column A

206. ______ V_A
207. ______ $\dot{V}O_2$
208. ______ $P_{A_{O_2}}$
209. ______ $\bar{P}CO_2$
210. ______ $F_{I_{O_2}}$
211. ______ DO_2
212. ______ $F_{I_{CO_2}}$
213. ______ V_E
214. ______ $\dot{V}_A$
215. ______ V_T
216. ______ V_D
217. ______ P_B

Column B

a. alveolar ventilation per minute
b. tidal volume
c. volume of deadspace gas
d. alveolar oxygen pressure
e. mean capillary oxygen pressure
f. volume of alveolar gas
g. barometric pressure
h. oxygen consumption per minute
i. volume of expired gas
j. diffusing capacity for oxygen
k. fractional concentration of carbon dioxide in inspired gas
l. fractional concentration of oxygen in inspired gas

Ref. 38, p. 330

In column A are listed the most frequently used symbols in pulmonary physiology for blood. In column B are listed the definitions of these symbols. Match column A with column B.

Column A

218. ______ Q
219. ______ $\dot{Q}$
220. ______ C
221. ______ S
222. ______ a
223. ______ v
224. ______ c

Column B

a. venous blood
b. capillary blood
c. volume of blood
d. concentration of gas in blood phase
e. % saturation of Hb with oxygen or carbon monoxide
f. arterial blood
g. volume flow of blood per unit time

Ref. 38, p. 331

In column A are listed some common examples frequently encountered in pulmonary physiology for blood. In column B are listed the definitions of these examples. Match column A with column B.

Column A

225. ______ Qc
226. ______ $\dot{Q}c$
227. ______ Pc_{CO}
228. ______ $S\bar{v}_{O_2}$
229. ______ Pa_{CO_2}
230. ______ $P\bar{v}_{O_2}$

Column B

a. partial pressure of CO_2 in arterial blood
b. partial pressure of O_2 in mixed venous blood
c. volume of blood in pulmonary capillaries
d. partial pressure of CO in pulmonary capillary blood
e. blood flow through pulmonary capillaries per minute
f. saturation of Hb with O_2 in mixed venous blood

Ref. 38, p. 331

SECTION 2

Evaluation Procedures, Methods and Techniques

For each of the questions select the *one* most appropriate answer.

231. To check the vital signs means to check:
a. pulse, blood pressure and heart rate
b. pulse, respiratory rate and heart rate
c. pulse, temperature and blood pressure
d. pulse, temperature and respiratory rate
e. pulse, blood pressure and respiratory rate

Ref. 7, p. 46

232. In which of the following arteries can a pulse not be felt?
a. brachial
b. dorsalis pedis
c. pulmonary
d. radial
e. carotid *Ref. 13, p. 460*

233. After taking the pulse of a child, the clinician should record the:
a. activity of the child at the time the pulse was taken
b. regularity or irregularity of rate
c. quality of pulse
d. rate
e. all of these *Ref. 40, p. 1068*

234. In a newborn infant the temperature should be taken:
a. orally
b. by axilla
c. rectally
d. all of these
e. a and c

Ref. 3, p. 89

235. The control of body temperature is called:
a. body heat
b. thermoinsulation
c. thermoregulation
d. thermal neutrality
e. thermal balance *Ref. 2, p. 50*

236. Loss of body heat in an infant may occur by:
a. convection
b. radiation
c. evaporation
d. conduction
e. all of these *Ref. 2, p. 59*

237. At birth a major cause of heat loss is:
a. convection
b. evaporation
c. radiation
d. conduction
e. osmosis *Ref. 2, p. 50*

238. In a preterm infant, a neutral thermal environment results in the:
a. least amount of body metabolism
b. lowest oxygen consumption
c. optimal caloric requirements
d. greatest comfort for the infant
e. none of these *Ref. 25, p. 38*

239. Evaporative heat loss in the delivery room is exaggerated by:
a. a wet baby
b. wet towels
c. air conditioning
d. all of these
e. a and c *Ref. 25, p. 39*

240. The normal axillary temperature of a newborn infant is:
a. 35 C
b. 36 C
c. 37 C
d. 38 C
e. 39 C *Ref. 41, p. 77*

241. If a child is having difficulty breathing, body temperature should be taken:

a. orally
b. by axilla
c. rectally
d. orally or by axilla
e. orally or rectally *Ref. 40, p. 1068*

242. Which of the following is the most accurate method of taking a patient's body temperature?

a. oral
b. axillary
c. rectal
d. there is no difference in accuracy
e. none of these *Ref. 42, p. 239*

243. In an infant, hyperthermia may be caused by:

a. sepsis
b. an overheated environment
c. antipyretics
d. all of these
e. a and b *Ref. 41, p. 77*

244. The effect that a decreased body temperature has on the oxygen-hemoglobin dissociation curve is:

a. the same as the effect of an increased pH
b. the curve shifts to the left
c. the oxygen % saturation is greater at any given PO_2
d. the oxygen becomes harder to remove from the hemoglobin
e. all of these *Ref. 12, p. 85*

245. The normal temperature in a newborn nursery is:

a. 60–65 F
b. 65–70 F
c. 70–75 F
d. 75–80 F
e. 80–85 F *Ref. 25, p. 39*

246. In regard to a patient's body temperature, which of the following is true?
a. rectal temperature is 1 F higher than oral
b. axillary temperature is 1 F higher than oral
c. rectal temperature is 1 F lower than oral
d. axillary temperature is equal to rectal temperature
e. none of these *Ref. 2, p. 61*

247. In a child, the body temperature should be taken rectally when the:
a. child has seizures
b. child has had oral surgery
c. child has difficulty breathing
d. child is receiving oxygen
e. all of these *Ref. 40, p. 1068*

248. Which of the following increases body temperature?
a. shock
b. exercise
c. cold drinks
d. bacterial invasion
e. b and d *Ref. 42, p. 239*

249. Rapid warming of a hypothermic infant may produce:
a. cyanosis
b. aspiration
c. apnea
d. retractions
e. stridor *Ref. 4, p. 91*

250. If an infant is chilled and restless instead of warm and quiet, what happens?
a. Pa_{O_2} increases
b. the anatomic deadspace-to-tidal volume ratio increases
c. metabolic rate increases
d. arterial carbon dioxide tensions increase
e. grunting and retractions start *Ref. 2, p. 61*

251. The normal respiratory rate for a sick newborn infant is:
a. 10–20 respirations per minute
b. 20–30 respirations per minute

c. 30–40 respirations per minute
d. 40–60 respirations per minute
e. over 60 respirations per minute *Ref. 4, p. 3*

252. A rapid respiratory rate in excess of metabolic needs with an increase in minute ventilation is termed:
a. hyperpnea
b. tachypnea
c. eupnea
d. bradypnea
e. oligopnea *Ref. 39, p. 306*

253. After counting the respiratory rate of a child, the clinician should record:
a. the rate and character of respirations
b. the activity of the child during observation
c. the color of the child
d. any signs of respiratory distress
e. all of these *Ref. 40, p. 1068*

254. The difference between the systolic pressure and the diastolic pressure is the:
a. blood pressure
b. central venous pressure
c. atrial pressure
d. pulse pressure
e. none of these *Ref. 11, p. 219*

255. The sounds heard over the artery when blood pressure is measured indirectly are:
a. Korotkoff sounds
b. hippocratic sounds
c. cardiac sounds
d. Santini's sounds
e. Winternitz's sounds *Ref. 43, p. 99*

256. The type of monitoring which provides an index of right atrial filling pressure and a guide to administration of blood and intravenous fluid is:

a. blood pressure
b. central venous pressure
c. pulse
d. heart rate
e. BUN *Ref. 44, pp. 128–30*

257. In regard to monitoring a patient's CVP, which of the following is true?

a. normal CVP is 5–10 cm/H_2O
b. a gradual rise or fall in CVP is more significant than an isolated value
c. mechanical ventilation causes a false, high CVP
d. vasopressors increase CVP
e. all of these *Ref. 44, pp. 128–30*

258. Excessive loss of fluids from the body results in states of:

a. restlessness
b. anxiety
c. dehydration
d. cyanosis
e. hypoxia *Ref. 9, p. 307*

259. The name of the scoring system commonly used to clinically evaluate infants at birth is:

a. Silverman-Andersen score
b. Apgar score
c. Miller score
d. Gregory score
e. RLF score *Ref. 2, p. 46*

260. The total score possible in the Apgar system is:

a. 4
b. 6
c. 8
d. 10
e. 12 *Ref. 2, p. 46*

261. The most important Apgar sign is:
a. heart rate
b. respiratory rate
c. muscle tone
d. reflex irritability
e. color *Ref. 45, p. 139*

262. At birth reflex irritability is judged by the infant's response to flicking the:
a. sole of the foot
b. fingers of the hand
c. kneecap
d. base of the chin
e. elbow *Ref. 2, pp. 47, 48*

263. The Apgar sign which refers to the degree of flexion and the resistance offered to straightening the extremities is:
a. heart rate
b. respiratory effort
c. muscle tone
d. reflex irritability
e. color *Ref. 2, p. 47*

264. Which of the following is not a component in the Apgar score?
a. heart rate
b. pulse
c. respiratory effort
d. muscle tone
e. color *Ref. 2, p. 47*

265. An Apgar score between 0 and 3 is an indication for:
a. suction
b. oxygen by bag and mask
c. intubation
d. closed chest massage
e. all of these *Ref. 25, pp. 34, 35*

266. An Apgar score of 4–6 signifies:
a. severe distress
b. moderate difficulty
c. absence of stress
d. no response
e. none of these *Ref. 2, p. 46*

267. The score which was developed for noting the breathing performance of premature infants based on signs of respiratory retraction is the:
a. Apgar score
b. Silverman-Andersen score
c. Miller score
d. Gregory score
e. RLF score *Ref. 46, p. 141*

268. Upon delivery the infant should not be stimulated by:
a. spanking
b. cold water showers
c. alternating hot and cold water baths
d. excessive rubbing of the back
e. any of these *Ref. 47, p. 16*

269. The delivery room care following the routine vaginal delivery of a healthy newborn does not include:
a. aspiration of the mouth and nose by a bulb syringe
b. maintenance of normal newborn temperature
c. routine identification procedures
d. cardiopulmonary resuscitation
e. silver nitrate ophthalmic prophylaxis
Ref. 47, p. 16

270. Immediately after delivery an infant is placed head down in the bassinet to:
a. increase venous return
b. allow gravity drainage of lung fluid
c. improve lung expansion
d. increase arterial oxygen levels
e. eliminate the tongue from obstructing the airway *Ref. 35, p. 204*

271. An infant who has a statistically increased chance of dying or becoming seriously compromised in the newborn period is considered:
a. premature
b. small for gestational age
c. high risk
d. large for gestational age
e. low birth weight *Ref. 33, p. 67*

272. The normal mode of breathing in the newborn is:
a. quiet
b. intercostal
c. diaphragmatic
d. labored
e. sternal *Ref. 17, p. 483*

273. Pyrexia is most closely related to:
a. pus
b. temperature
c. pressure
d. infection
e. umbilical catheterization *Ref. 1, p. 1051*

274. If insertion of an oropharyngeal airway causes the patient to cough, swallow, gag or vomit, the clinician should:
a. remove the airway and hyperextend the head
b. quickly tape the airway and use suction
c. remove the airway and turn the head to the side
d. remove the airway and use suction
e. none of these *Ref. 48, p. 36*

275. Endotracheal tube connectors are regulated by:
a. N.F.P.A.
b. American National Standards Institute
c. Compressed Gas Association
d. Interstate Commerce Commission
e. Department of Transportation *Ref. 49, p. 307*

276. The purpose of a stylet is to:
a. suction the nasopharynx and oropharynx
b. help direct the tracheal tube through the vocal cords
c. keep the patient from biting the tube
d. increase the curvature of the tracheal tube
e. connect the tube to an ancillary device

Ref. 48, p. 42

277. What part of an endotracheal tube can cause pressure necrosis?
a. inflating tube
b. pilot balloon
c. bevel
d. cuff
e. adapter *Ref. 26, p. 361*

278. Which of the following statements about laryngoscopes are true?
a. a laryngoscope is composed of a blade, handle and light
b. each blade is composed of a spatula, flange and tip
c. the difference between a McIntosh and Miller blade is in the construction of the spatula
d. the blade tip elevates the epiglottis
e. all of these *Ref. 49, pp. 298–302*

279. When a pharyngeal airway is inserted into the mouth of an infant the purpose is:
a. to hold the tongue away from the anterior pharyngeal wall
b. to hold the tongue away from the posterior pharyngeal wall
c. to hold the tongue forward from the soft palate
d. a and c
e. b and c *Ref. 46, p. 152*

280. A nasopharyngeal airway is preferred over an oropharyngeal airway in children with:
a. temporomandibular joint immobility
b. convulsions
c. facial trauma

d. all of these
e. a and c *Ref. 4, p. 138*

281. The insertion of a nasopharyngeal airway in children can cause:
a. epistaxis
b. laryngospasm
c. regurgitation
d. convulsions
e. respiratory depression *Ref. 4, p. 136*

282. Which of the following airways is best suited for use in children?
a. Berman
b. Brook
c. Guedel
d. all of these
e. a and b *Ref. 4, p. 137*

283. The airway of choice in an infant with bilateral choanal atresia is a:
a. nasopharyngeal airway
b. oropharyngeal airway
c. nasotracheal tube
d. orotracheal tube
e. tracheostomy tube *Ref. 41, p. 84*

284. An S tube is used to:
a. intubate the airway
b. ventilate the patient
c. suction the patient
d. provide mechanical external compression
e. none of these *Ref. 48, p. 36*

285. Nasotracheal intubation is contraindicated in:
a. nasal obstruction
b. nasal infection
c. nasal inflammation
d. all of these
e. none of these *Ref. 41, p. 105*

286. Small, premature infants use a nasotracheal tube with a:
a. 2.5 mm O.D.
b. 2.5 mm I.D.
c. 3.0 mm O.D.
d. 3.0 mm I.D.
e. 3.5 mm O.D. *Ref. 50, p. 355*

287. The most common size nasotracheal tube used in newborn infants is:
a. 2.5 mm
b. 3.0 mm
c. 3.5 mm
d. 4.0 mm
e. 4.5 mm *Ref. 51, p. 242*

288. In which size nasotracheal tube is resistance to flow the greatest?
a. 4.0 mm
b. 4.5 mm
c. 5.0 mm
d. 6.5 mm
e. 8.0 mm *Ref. 51, p. 242*

289. In which of the following nasotracheal tube sizes is suctioning most difficult?
a. 2.5 mm
b. 3.0 mm
c. 3.5 mm
d. 4.0 mm
e. 4.5 mm *Ref. 51, p. 242*

290. Which of these factors is not responsible for complications in nasotracheal intubation?
a. size of the tube
b. silicone composition of the tube
c. trauma at the time of intubation
d. the pneumatic piston effect of the ventilator
e. the duration of intubation *Ref. 51, p. 241*

291. When seen by radiography, a nasotracheal tube should lie:
a. about the level of the medial ends of the clavicles
b. at the eighth cartilaginous ring

c. just above the carina
d. near the bifurcation of the right main stem bronchus
e. near the bifurcation of the left main stem bronchus *Ref. 41, p. 106*

292. Intubation of the neonate is accomplished by using:
a. an uncuffed tube
b. a cuffed tube
c. a mask cemented to the neonate's face for better ventilation, rather than a tube
d. none of these
e. all of these *Ref. 4, p. 145*

293. In infants and small children, the largest size endotracheal tube should be inserted to:
a. minimize damage to the mucosa by excessive motion
b. reduce the air leaks around the tube
c. minimize the possibility of increased airway resistance
d. all of these
e. a and b *Ref. 52, p. 128*

294. The least-used indication for endotracheal intubation is to:
a. maintain a patent airway
b. permit mechanical ventilation
c. decrease anatomical deadspace
d. prevent aspiration
e. facilitate removal of secretions *Ref. 53, p. 51*

295. A Cole tube does *not*:
a. help prevent endobronchial intubation
b. allow large adapters to be used
c. facilitate suctioning
d. increase gas flow resistance
e. seal off the glottic opening *Ref. 24, p. 136*

296. The advantages of the Cole tube are:
a. lower resistance
b. larger resistance
c. less likelihood of endobronchial intubation
d. a and c
e. b and c *Ref. 54, p. 250*

297. The length of the Cole tube is usually between:

a. 1.0–1.5 cm
b. 2.0–2.5 cm
c. 2.5–4.5 cm
d. 4.5–6.0 cm
e. 6.0–8.0 cm *Ref. 54, p. 250*

298. Cole tubes are sized according to:

a. I.D.
b. O.D.
c. I.D. of the smaller bore intratracheal portion
d. O.D. of the smaller bore intratracheal portion
e. none of these *Ref. 54, p. 250*

299. A disadvantage of the Cole tube is that it:

a. cannot be used nasally
b. increases resistance
c. often results in endobronchial intubation
d. cannot be used in pediatrics
e. reduces deadspace *Ref. 54, p. 250*

300. The most frequent error resulting from too deep an introduction of the laryngoscope into the infant pharynx is.

a. trauma to the pharynx
b. intubation of the esophagus
c. intubation of the right main stem bronchus
d. infection
e. intubation of the left main stem bronchus

Ref. 46, p. 163

301. In infants the tip of the endotracheal tube should be inserted how far below the level of the vocal cords?

a. 0.5 cm
b. 1.0 cm
c. 2.0 cm
d. 1 in.
e. 1–2 in. *Ref. 55, p. 315*

302. Which of the following areas should never be traumatized during endotracheal intubation?

a. pharynx

b. epiglottis
c. aryepiglottic folds
d. vocal cords
e. all of these *Ref. 46, p. 163*

303. Noncuffed endotracheal tubes are used for children up to ______ kg in weight.
a. 10
b. 15
c. 20
d. 25
e. 30 *Ref. 24, p. 143*

304. Children usually require a cuffed endotracheal tube at age:
a. 6 years
b. 8 years
c. 10 years
d. 12 years
e. 14 years *Ref. 36, p. 14*

305. Cuffs should not be used on endotracheal tubes less than:
a. 4.0 mm
b. 5.0 mm
c. 6.0 mm
d. 6.5 mm
e. 7.0 mm *Ref. 24, p. 136*

306. An endotracheal or tracheostomy tube cuff is used primarily to:
a. stabilize the tube
b. provide a closed breathing circuit
c. prevent trauma to the walls of the trachea by acting as a cushion around the tube
d. eliminate talking
e. provide effective mechanical ventilation

Ref. 26, p. 353

307. Overinflation of an endotracheal or tracheostomy tube cuff for a long period of time will usually result in:

a. a vocal loss after removal of the tube
b. a gag reflex
c. tracheal tissue snowplowing
d. tracheal necrosis
e. all of these *Ref. 26, p. 361*

308. What is the major reason for deflating a cuff on a ventilator patient?

a. to prevent aspiration
b. to allow hyperoxygenation
c. to prevent aspiration
d. to prevent tracheal necrosis
e. to listen for breath sounds *Ref. 26, p. 361*

309. If an endotracheal tube which is too large for a child is used, what complications can occur?

a. edema
b. pressure necrosis
c. bronchial intubation
d. all of these
e. b and c *Ref. 4, p. 145*

310. If breath sounds or chest excursions are not equal bilaterally following endotracheal intubation, you should:

a. push the tube in a little farther
b. immediately extubate the patient
c. pull the tube back slightly
d. take a chest x-ray
e. manually bag the patient *Ref. 55, p. 316*

311. Following intubation, placement of the endotracheal tube should be checked by:

a. rise and fall of the chest
b. chest radiography
c. auscultation
d. all of these
e. b and c *Ref. 53, p. 53*

312. Following endotracheal intubation, if the clinician hears breath sounds over the stomach and/or sees stomach distention, it generally means the tube is:
a. in the right main stem bronchus
b. in the left main stem bronchus
c. at the carina
d. in the esophagus
e. any of these *Ref. 33, p. 21*

313. The introduction of an endotracheal tube in an infant with hyaline membrane disease abolishes:
a. tachypnea
b. cyanosis
c. grunting
d. retractions
e. secretions *Ref. 32, p. 155*

314. If, after endotracheal intubation, the epigastrium rises and the chest does not, the most likely conclusion is:
a. the tube is in the right main stem bronchus
b. the tube is in the left main stem bronchus
c. the tube is at the carina
d. the tube is in the esophagus
e. all of these are possibilities *Ref. 46, p. 163*

315. The purpose of a chest roentgenogram following endotracheal intubation is to:
a. evaluate the disease process
b. ascertain laryngeal damage
c. prevent lateral wall erosion
d. exclude bronchial intubation
e. check for mediastinal shifts *Ref. 36, p. 14*

316. Cuffed endotracheal tubes are never necessary in infants and small children because the:
a. cricoid diameter is narrow
b. thyroid isthmus is larger than in adults
c. transverse diameter of the glottis is reduced
d. larynx is immature
e. tracheal length is so small *Ref. 36, p. 14*

317. Which of the following can be considered an artificial airway?
a. pharyngeal tube
b. nasotracheal tube
c. endotracheal tube
d. tracheostomy tube
e. all of these *Ref. 56, pp. 15, 16*

318. Which of the following is not a potential complication of tracheal airways?
a. displacement
b. occlusion
c. breakage
d. infection
e. impaction *Ref. 36, p. 15*

319. At an age of less than 1 month, it is dangerous to perform a tracheotomy because:
a. of the small size of the trachea
b. infections are common
c. the tracheal cartilages are soft and this procedure could cause the trachea to collapse after removal of the tube
d. tube displacement often occurs
e. all of these *Ref. 57, p. 159*

320. Once a patient has been tracheotomized, the anatomical deadspace usually:
a. increases
b. decreases
c. remains unchanged
d. is abolished
e. none of these *Ref. 26, p. 357*

321. Which of the following is not an indication for tracheotomy in children?
a. to reduce anatomical deadspace
b. to decrease lung compliance
c. to facilitate suctioning of the airway
d. to bypass obstruction of the upper airway
e. to facilitate prolonged mechanical ventilation *Ref. 4, p. 155*

322. Clinical evidence of hypoxia in the newborn includes:
a. pallor and cyanosis
b. tachycardia
c. tachypnea
d. abdominal distention
e. all of these *Ref. 25, p. 45*

323. A sound made by an infant exhaling against a partially closed glottis is called:
a. retractions
b. tachypnea
c. grunting
d. cyanosis
e. hyperpnea *Ref. 25, p. 48*

324. In the first hour of life a normal infant may have:
a. tachypnea
b. rales
c. grunting
d. all of these
e. a and b *Ref. 33, p. 105*

325. After the first hour of life the normal infant should not have:
a. retractions
b. rales
c. grunting
d. all of these
e. a and c *Ref. 33, p. 105*

326. Stridor is most closely related to:
a. disease
b. obstruction
c. dilation
d. cyanosis
e. elasticity *Ref. 33, p. 105*

327. The phenomenon grunting:
a. is due to poor perfusion
b. increases the transpulmonary pressure
c. is due to progressive collapse of alveoli
d. occurs when hemoglobin is reduced 5 vol %
e. is synonymous with retractions *Ref. 32, p. 155*

328. Which of the following signs are indications of respiratory distress in the newborn?
a. grunting
b. retractions
c. nasal flaring
d. tachypnea
e. all of these *Ref. 25, p. 48*

329. Respiratory distress is present in the neonate when the respiratory rate is above:
a. 30 breaths per minute
b. 40 breaths per minute
c. 50 breaths per minute
d. 60 breaths per minute
e. 70 breaths per minute *Ref. 4, p. 3*

330. If severe enough, hypoxemia becomes clinically apparent as visible:
a. grunting
b. retractions
c. cyanosis
d. tachycardia
e. eupnea *Ref. 34, p. 17*

331. Infants born moderately or severely depressed are:
a. infants with low Apgar scores
b. infants with meconium-stained amniotic fluid
c. infants with history of fetal distress
d. infants delivered by emergency cesarean section
e. all of these *Ref. 33, p. 67*

332. A clinical sign of small airway narrowing is:
a. cyanosis
b. wheezing
c. tachycardia
d. bradypnea
e. hyperthermia *Ref. 39, pp. 314, 315*

333. Which of the following decreases the range of expansion of the lung?
a. grunting
b. wheezing

c. retractions
d. nasal flaring
e. inspiration *Ref. 39, p. 308*

334. Which of the following cannot be diagnosed through visual clinical evaluation?
a. retractions
b. cyanosis
c. acidosis
d. grunting
e. nasal flaring *Ref. 25, p. 35*

335. One of the effects of upper respiratory obstruction is:
a. grunting
b. stridor
c. cyanosis
d. eupnea
e. nasal flaring *Ref. 39, p. 311*

336. The science of reanimatology is the study of:
a. endotracheal intubation
b. bronchoscopy
c. resuscitation
d. arterial puncture
e. mechanical ventilation *Ref. 58, p. 3*

337. Cessation of breathing and circulation is the definition of:
a. asphyxia
b. clinical death
c. biological death
d. cardiac arrest
e. respiratory arrest *Ref. 59, p. 4*

338. An example of a respiratory arrest would be:
a. massive hemorrhage
b. complete airway obstruction
c. digitalis toxicity
d. cardiac catheterization
e. pulmonary embolism *Ref. 59, p. 19*

339. An example of a circulatory arrest would be:
a. neuromuscular paralysis
b. oxygen deprivation
c. ventricular fibrillation
d. chemical poisoning
e. overdose of sedatives *Ref. 59, p. 19*

340. The most reliable clinical signs of cardiac arrest are:
a. absence of breathing
b. absence of carotid or femoral pulse
c. dilation of pupils
d. all of these
e. a and b *Ref. 59, pp. 4–6*

341. If enlarged pupils do not become smaller with prompt resuscitation, it usually means:
a. the resuscitation is ineffective
b. resuscitation was significantly delayed
c. that there may be brain damage which is not necessarily permanent
d. all of these
e. b and c *Ref. 59, pp. 7, 8, 105*

342. The carotid pulse is best felt by deep palpation between the thyroid cartilage and the anterior edge of the:
a. styloid process
b. carotid artery
c. sternocleidomastoid muscle
d. mandible
e. none of these *Ref. 60, p. 5*

343. If you can palpate a carotid pulse during CPR, it is an indication of:
a. adequate pressure
b. adequate flow
c. adequate output
d. none of these
e. a and b *Ref. 59, p. 105*

344. The most common circumstances that result in the need for neonatal resuscitation are:

a. meconium aspiration
b. prolapsed cord
c. toxemia of pregnancy
d. emergency cesarean section
e. all of these *Ref. 61, p. 69*

345. The two most important steps in cardiopulmonary resuscitation are:

a. opening the airway
b. hyperextending the neck
c. restoring breathing
d. a and b
e. a and c *Ref. 62, p. 841*

346. The frequency of mouth-to-mouth resuscitation in an infant is:

a. 10–20 breaths per minute
b. 20–35 breaths per minute
c. 35–45 breaths per minute
d. 45–60 breaths per minute
e. 60–80 breaths per minute *Ref. 62, p. 843*

347. Which of the following can be considered a method of artificial ventilation?

a. mouth to mouth
b. mouth to nose
c. mouth to S tube
d. mouth to non-rebreathing valve
e. all of these *Ref. 62, pp. 842, 853*

348. The most common method of emergency artificial ventilation in infants and small children is:

a. mouth to mouth
b. mouth to nose
c. mouth to nose and mouth
d. mouth to S tube
e. mouth to pharyngeal airway *Ref. 59, p. 51*

349. Adequate mouth-to-mouth ventilation is determined on every breath by:
a. adequate rise of the chest
b. hearing air escape during exhalation
c. feeling a femoral pulse
d. all of these
e. a and c *Ref. 59, p. 46*

350. During resuscitation, the most efficacious concentration of oxygen is:
a. 21%–40%
b. 40%
c. 50%–70%
d. 70%–90%
e. 100% *Ref. 59, p. 56*

351. The expired air of a hyperventilating operator contains about ______ less oxygen than ambient air.
a. 3%–5%
b. 2%–3%
c. 4%–6%
d. 1%
e. 5% *Ref. 59, p. 46*

352. The jaw relaxes in an unconscious patient and allows the tongue to fall back and meet the ______, thus obstructing the airway.
a. anterior pharynx
b. anterior larynx
c. posterior pharynx
d. posterior larynx
e. none of these *Ref. 59, p. 26*

353. External cardiac massage in an infant should be at a rate of:
a. 20–40 per minute
b. 40–60 per minute
c. 60–80 per minute
d. 80–100 per minute
e. 100–120 per minute *Ref. 62, p. 846*

354. In an infant or small child, external cardiac compression is applied to the:
a. first third of the sternum
b. midportion of the sternum
c. lower third of the sternum
d. manubrium
e. xiphoid process *Ref. 62, p. 846*

355. The most common complication of external cardiac massage in children is:
a. fracture of the manubrium
b. liver laceration
c. rib fracture
d. pneumothorax
e. none of these *Ref. 62, p. 846*

356. Which of the following is not a possible complication of external cardiac massage?
a. fracture of the sternum
b. rib fracture
c. innominate artery erosion
d. damage to the liver
e. damage to the spleen *Ref. 62, p. 68*

357. In infants requiring external cardiac massage, the sternum should be depressed:
a. ¼ in.
b. ¼–½in.
c. ½–¾ in.
d. ¾–1 in.
e. 1–1¼ in. *Ref. 62, p. 846*

358. In children requiring external cardiac massage, the sternum should be depressed:
a. ¼ in.
b. ¼–1 in.
c. ½–1 in.
d. ¾–1½ in.
e. 1½–3 in. *Ref. 62, p. 846*

359. External cardiac massage is performed on infants by:
a. using the fingers of the hand
b. using the tips of the index and middle finger
c. using the thumb and forefinger
d. using the heel of the hand
e. none of these *Ref. 62, p. 846*

360. During properly applied cardiac compression, cardiac output is about _____ of normal.
a. 5%–15%
b. 15%–30%
c. 30%–50%
d. 50%–70%
e. 70%–90% *Ref. 59, p. 61*

361. During cardiopulmonary resuscitation, the signs of adequate cardiac output are:
a. improvement in color
b. constriction of pupils
c. palpable arterial pulses
d. all of these
e. a and c *Ref. 35, p. 208*

362. The most important factor contributing to a successful resuscitation is the:
a. cause of death
b. volume of ventilation
c. depth of cardiac massage
d. immediate opening of the airway
e. number of cardiac compressions

Ref. 53, p. 284

363. Immediate resuscitative measures do not include:
a. aspiration of upper airway secretions
b. manual ventilation with a bag and mask
c. administration of bicarbonate
d. tracheal intubation
e. mechanical ventilation *Ref. 35, p. 240*

364. Specific indications for open-chest cardiac massage are:
a. trauma to the thoracic cage
b. perforating thoracic injuries

c. the likelihood of a tension pneumothorax
d. all of these
e. a and b *Ref. 59, p. 73*

365. An electrocardiogram:
a. is a guide to the electrical activity of the heart
b. reveals the effectiveness of the heart as a pump
c. should be obtained if at all possible during resuscitation
d. all of these
e. a and c *Ref. 59, p. 85*

366. The ECG pattern in asystole looks like:
a. an erratic pattern
b. a straight line
c. a fast up-and-down motion of even shape
d. all of these
e. none of these *Ref. 59, p. 87*

367. The ECG pattern in fibrillation looks like:
a. an erratic pattern
b. a straight line
c. a fast up-and-down motion of even shape
d. all of these
e. none of these *Ref. 59, p. 88*

368. Cardiac output during fibrillation is:
a. zero
b. 20% of normal
c. 40% of normal
d. 60% of normal
e. 80% of normal *Ref. 59, p. 89*

369. Bicarbonate therapy is indicated after cardiac arrest to:
a. eliminate acidosis
b. reduce myocardial contractility
c. increase myocardial contractility
d. a and b
e. a and c *Ref. 36, p. 5*

370. Epinephrine is used in cardiac resuscitation to:
a. increase the head pressure of cardiac compression
b. relieve bronchospasm
c. stimulate the myocardium
d. stop fibrillation
e. a and c *Ref. 59, p. 79*

371. During cardiac arrest, metabolic acidosis is caused by an accumulation or a build-up of:
a. pyruvic acid
b. lactic acid
c. oxalic acid
d. all of these
e. a and b *Ref. 60, p. 114*

372. An adequate resuscitation bag-valve-mask unit should:
a. be self-refilling
b. provide high oxygen concentrations
c. possess a 15/22 mm fitting
d. all of these
e. a and b *Ref. 62, p. 853*

373. A potential problem not associated with the use of a bag and mask for ventilation is:
a. corneal laceration
b. overventilation
c. underventilation
d. hypocapnia
e. tracheal ischemia *Ref. 55, p. 314*

374. Some possible complications arising from the use of bag-and-mask units in an infant are:
a. pressure necrosis
b. gastric distention
c. pneumothorax
d. all of these
e. a and b *Ref. 25, p. 122*

375. The purpose of a bleed hole in an infant manual resuscitation device is to:
a. increase the feel
b. reduce the recoil time

c. prevent rebreathing
d. limit the pressure
e. none of these *Ref. 63, p. 243*

376. The purpose of a reservoir tube on a self-inflating resuscitation device is to:
a. prevent rebreathing
b. serve as a mechanical pop-off
c. increase the FI_{O_2}
d. decrease the inflation pressure
e. increase the bag capacity *Ref. 59, p. 57*

377. Which of these self-inflating resuscitation bags have a reservoir tube?
a. Laerdal
b. Cardiff Infant Inflating Bag
c. Hope Pediatric
d. a and b
e. a and c *Refs. 60, p. 26; 4, p. 162*

378. Which of these self-inflating resuscitation bags have a pop-off valve?
a. Cardiff Infant inflating bag
b. PMR
c. Hope Pediatric
d. a and b
e. a and c *Refs. 64–66*

379. Which adult hand-resuscitation device also has a pediatric counterpart with a magnetic pop-off?
a. PMR
b. Hope
c. Ambu
d. Penlon
e. none of these *Refs. 65–69*

380. The capacity of the Cardiff Infant inflating bag is:
a. 50 ml
b. 100 ml
c. 150 ml
d. 250 ml
e. 125 ml *Ref. 64*

381. The capacity of the reservoir tube on the Cardiff Infant inflating bag is:
a. 30 ml
b. 50 ml
c. 80 ml
d. 100 ml
e. 125 ml *Ref. 64*

382. The Hope Pediatric resuscitation device has what capacity?
a. 780 ml
b. 750 ml
c. 730 ml
d. 800 ml
e. 500 ml *Ref. 66*

383. The difference between the adult and pediatric Hope resuscitation devices is that the pediatric device has a valve assembly with a:
a. shorter stroke and quicker response time
b. shorter stroke and longer response time
c. longer stroke and longer response time
d. longer stroke and shorter response time
e. none of these *Refs. 66, 68*

384. In the Hope Pediatric resuscitation device an optional pop-off valve of ______ cm H_2O is available.
a. 20
b. 30
c. 40
d. 50
e. 60 *Ref. 66*

385. A postural drainage technique based on the anatomic structure of the tracheobronchial tree and the effect of gravity is:
a. coughing
b. percussion
c. positioning
d. vibration
e. segmental breathing *Ref. 25, p. 137*

386. A method of chest physical therapy performed with a cupped hand is:

a. coughing
b. percussion
c. positioning
d. vibration
e. segmental breathing *Ref. 25, p. 142*

387. Contraindications to the use of percussion are:

a. fractures of the ribs
b. hemoptysis
c. excessive pain
d. all of these
e. none of these *Ref. 25, p. 143*

388. A method of physical therapy characterized by a fine, shaking motion achieved by tightening the muscles of the upper extremities and shoulder girdle is:

a. coughing
b. percussion
c. positioning
d. vibration
e. segmental breathing *Ref. 25, p. 143*

389. A routine chest examination includes all of the following except:

a. palpation
b. auscultation
c. inspection
d. palpitation
e. percussion *Ref. 70, pp. 232–47*

In column A are listed the various segments requiring postural drainage. In column B are listed the various postural drainage positions. Match column A with column B.

Column A

390. _____ upper lobe, apical bronchus

391. _____ upper lobe, right posterior bronchus

392. _____ upper lobe, left posterior bronchus

393. _____ upper lobe, anterior bronchus

394. _____ middle lobe, lateral and medial bronchus

395. _____ lingula, superior and inferior bronchus

396. _____ lower lobe, apical bronchus

397. _____ right medial basal bronchus

398. _____ anterior basal bronchus

399. _____ right lateral basal bronchus

400. _____ posterior basal bronchus

Column B

a. lying flat on bed with knees slightly flexed

b. lying flat on back, body quarter-turned to left maintained by a pillow under right side from shoulder to hip, foot of bed raised 14 in.

c. lying flat on back, buttocks resting on a pillow and knees flexed, foot of bed raised 18 in.

d. lying flat on face with a pillow under the hips, foot of bed raised 18 in.

e. sitting upright with slight variations according to position

f. lying flat on face, pillow under the hips

g. lying on left side horizontally, and then turned 45 degrees onto face, resting against a pillow, with another supporting the head

h. lying on left side, foot of bed raised 18 in., a pillow under the hips

i. lying on right side, turned 45 degrees onto face with 3 pillows arranged to lift shoulders 12 in.

j. lying flat on back, body quarter-turned to right maintained by a pillow under left side from shoulder to hip, foot of bed raised 14 in.
k. lying on right side, foot of bed raised 18 in., a pillow under the hips

Ref. 18, pp. 13–15

401. Postural drainage can be given to infants and small children by placing them over the clinician's:
a. bed
b. arm
c. abdomen
d. knee
e. stomach

Ref. 18, p. 12

402. The aim of breathing exercises is to:
a. promote a normal, relaxed pattern of breathing
b. assist with removal of secretions
c. teach controlled breathing
d. all of these
e. a and b

Ref. 18, p. 5

403. Postural drainage has been ordered following aerosol-IPPB therapy for a cystic fibrosis patient. Which of the following positions would you employ to drain the upper lobe apical bronchus?
a. prone
b. left lateral decubitus
c. supine
d. head and chest down toward the floor at an angle of 45 degrees
e. none of these

Ref. 18, p. 13

In column A are listed several terms relating to cleaning and sterilization. In column B are listed several definitions. Match column A to column B.

Column A

404. ______ bacteria
405. ______ spore
406. ______ virus
407. ______ sterilization
408. ______ disinfection
409. ______ antiseptic
410. ______ bactericide
411. ______ bacteriostat
412. ______ sanitation
413. ______ decontamination

Column B

a. reduction of the number of bacteria to safe levels
b. a process which destroys all vegetative bacteria but not spores
c. an agent which kills bacteria
d. infectious agents smaller in size than bacteria
e. any substance that has a bactericidal or bacteriostatic effect and can be safely applied to the skin
f. the normal resting stage in the life cycle of certain bacteria
g. minute unicellular organisms which usually multiply by binary division
h. destruction of all forms of microorganisms
i. the elimination of a harmful substance
j. an agent which will prevent bacterial growth but does not necessarily kill the bacteria

Ref. 54

414. Sterilization can best be defined as:
- a. the complete destruction of all microorganisms except spores
- b. an agent that impedes the growth of bacteria but does not kill them
- c. an agent that destroys all living bacteria and impedes the growth of spores
- d. the complete destruction or removal of all viable microorganisms
- e. none of these *Ref. 71, p. 105*

415. In steam sterilization the pressurized steam works by:
- a. alkylation
- b. denaturing microbial proteins through heat and coagulation
- c. forming nonviable compounds
- d. denaturing proteins and forming a substance called ethylene glycol
- e. none of these *Ref. 72, p. 10*

416. Another name for CIDEX is which of the following?
- a. glutaraldehyde
- b. activated dialdehyde
- c. activated glutaraldehyde
- d. a and b
- e. b and c *Refs. 73, p. 458; 54, p. 287*

417. The active ingredient in CIDEX is which of the following?
- a. dialdehyde
- b. bicarbonate
- c. glutaraldehyde
- d. sodium bisulfate
- e. none of these *Ref. 73, p. 458*

418. Because CIDEX loses its effectiveness after a certain period of time, it should be changed every:
- a. 12 days
- b. 2 weeks
- c. 10 days
- d. 14 days
- e. b and d *Ref. 73, p. 459*

419. In 10 hours CIDEX can be classified as:
a. bactericidal
b. pseudomonocidal
c. virucidal
d. sporicidal
e. all of these *Ref. 54, p. 287*

420. In 10 minutes CIDEX acts as which of the following agents:
a. bactericidal
b. tuberculocidal
c. pseudomonocidal
d. virucidal
e. all of these *Ref. 54, p. 287*

421. Autoclaving is:
a. moist heat in the form of saturated steam
b. moist heat in the form of saturated steam under pressure
c. readily accomplished at 100 F
d. a sterilizing process which kills everything except spores
e. the method of choice for sterilizing heat-sensitive materials *Ref. 54, p. 285*

422. Another name for autoclaving is:
a. heat-steam sterilization
b. CIDEX
c. gas sterilization
d. ethylene oxide
e. pasteurization *Ref. 25, p. 184*

423. The chemical formula of ethylene oxide is:
a. $(CH_2)O_2$
b. $(CH_2)O$
c. $(CH_2)_2O$
d. $(CH_2)O_2H$
e. $(CH_2)_2OH$

Ref. 74, p. 160

424. The lethal action of ethylene oxide depends upon:
a. the concentration of the gas in contact with the microorganisms
b. temperature
c. relative humidity
d. duration of exposure
e. all of these *Ref. 75*

425. Which of the following concentrations of ethylene oxide are explosive?
a. 12% ETO/88% Freon 12
b. 12% ETO/88% Ucon 12
c. 10% ETO/90% CO_2
d. 100% ETO
e. all are explosive *Ref. 75*

426. Polyethylene is commonly used as a wrapping in ETO sterilization because:
a. ethylene oxide passes through very easily
b. it is not used as a wrapping
c. it hinders elution
d. a and c
e. none of these *Ref. 54, p. 289*

427. All of the following are advantages of ethylene oxide sterilization except:
a. reliability
b. wide applicability of use
c. minimal damage to equipment
d. short-term storage
e. ability to prepackage equipment
Ref. 54, p. 288

428. The major hazards of ethylene oxide are:
a. inadequate poststerilization aeration
b. skin reactions
c. laryngotracheal inflammation
d. all of these
e. a and b *Ref. 54, p. 289*

429. Any polyvinylchloride substances sterilized by gamma irradiation should never be sterilized by ETO because:

a. it may form ethylene chlorhydrin
b. it may form ethylene glycol
c. the equipment may cause burns when used on patients
d. a and c
e. b and c *Ref. 54, p. 289*

430. Which of the following should never be used for wrapping equipment which is to be ethylene-oxide sterilized?

a. polypropylene
b. paper wrap
c. cloth
d. all of these can be used
e. none of these *Ref. 54, p. 289*

431. Ethylene oxide plus water forms:

a. ethylene glycol
b. ethylene chlorhydrin
c. ethylene oxide
d. ethylene dioxide
e. ethylene chloride *Ref. 54, p. 289*

SECTION 3

Acid-Base Chemistry, Arterial Blood Gases and Pharmacology

For each of the following questions select the *one* most appropriate answer.

432. A cation is:
- a. a neutral ion
- b. a negatively charged ion
- c. a positively charged ion
- d. an ion with a deficit of electrons
- e. an ion with no electrical charge *Ref. 28, p. 46*

433. An anion is:
- a. a neutral ion
- b. a negatively charged ion
- c. a positively charged ion
- d. an ion with no electrical charge
- e. none of these *Ref. 28, p. 46*

434. The principal cation in interstitial fluid is:
- a. chloride
- b. sodium
- c. potassium
- d. bicarbonate
- e. magnesium *Ref. 9, p. 304*

435. The principal anions of interstitial fluid are:
- a. sodium and potassium
- b. chloride and sodium
- c. potassium and bicarbonate
- d. bicarbonate and sodium
- e. chloride and bicarbonate *Ref. 9, p. 304*

436. According to the Bronsted theory, a substance which can donate hydrogen ions is:
a. a buffer
b. an acid
c. a base
d. an anion
e. a solute *Ref. 76, p. 1*

437. Also according to the Bronsted theory, a substance which can accept hydrogen ions is:
a. an acid
b. a base
c. a bicarbonate
d. a cation
e. a solute *Ref. 76, p. 1*

438. The symbol used to describe the hydrogen ion concentration of the body is:
a. H_2CO_3
b. pH
c. HCO_3^-
d. C.O.
e. PB *Ref. 28, p. 48*

439. The term pH equals:
a. log H^+ concentration
b. log $1/[H^+]$
c. $-\log [H^+]$
d. a and b
e. b and c *Ref. 11, p. 427*

440. The pK of the bicarbonate buffer system at BTPS is:
a. 6.1
b. 7.0
c. 7.4
d. 8.0
e. 9.0 *Ref. 11, p. 429*

441. The pK is the pH at which the substance is:
a. dissociated
b. undissociated
c. half dissociated and half undissociated

d. acidotic
e. alkalotic *Ref. 28, p. 48*

442. The logarithm of 20 is:
a. 1.0
b. 1.1
c. 1.2
d. 1.3
e. 1.4 *Ref. 28, p. 48*

443. The entire range of pH is:
a. 0–7
b. 7.35–7.45
c. 0–14
d. 7.38–7.42
e. 0–10 *Ref. 26, p. 54*

444. The range of physiological pH is:
a. 0–7
b. 0–14
c. 6.8–8.0
d. 7.0–7.8
e. 0–8 *Ref. 12, p. 109*

445. The blood pH of normal newborn infants varies between:
a. 7.40–7.52
b. 7.35–7.44
c. 7.38–7.47
d. 7.30–7.50
e. 7.25–7.50 *Ref. 9, p. 305*

446. The normal range of pH in children is:
a. 7.40
b. 7.38–7.42
c. 7.34–7.44
d. 7.32–7.42
e. 7.40–7.50 *Ref. 9, p. 305*

447. What values must be known to determine arterial pH indirectly?

a. H_2CO_3 and Pa_{CO_2}
b. Pa_{CO_2} and pK
c. HCO_3 and Pa_{CO_2}
d. H_2CO_3 and pK
e. HCO_3 and pK *Ref. 77, p. 57*

448. $H_2O + CO_2$ yields:

a. HCO_3
b. $NaHCO_3$
c. H_2CO_3
d. $CO_3 + H^+$
e. none of these *Ref. 76, p. 15*

449. The formation of H_2CO_3 from CO_2 and H_2O:

a. is catalyzed by carbonic hydrase
b. occurs rapidly without a catalyst
c. is catalyzed by an enzyme present in red blood cells
d. takes place in the kidneys only
e. none of these *Ref. 28, p. 50*

Match the following acid-base disorders with their description:

450. ______ an acidosis which is reflected by a decrease of standard bicarbonate
451. ______ the result of a decreased Pa_{CO_2}
452. ______ an alkalosis which is reflected by an increase of standard bicarbonate
453. ______ the result of an increased Pa_{CO_2}

a. respiratory acidosis
b. respiratory alkalosis
c. metabolic acidosis
d. metabolic alkalosis
Ref. 12, p. 116

454. The equation $pH = pK + \log \frac{[HCO_3]}{[H_2CO_3]}$ was first described by:

a. Henderson
b. Hasselbalch
c. Henderson-Hasselbalch
d. Boyle
e. Charles *Ref. 26, p. 115*

In column A are listed various acid-base symbols or terms. In column B are listed the definitions. Match column A and column B.

Column A

455. ______ acid
Ref. 28, p. 187

456. ______ anion
Ref. 28, p. 188

457. ______ base
Ref. 28, p. 187

458. ______ acidemia
Ref. 28, p. 187

459. ______ alkalemia
Ref. 28, p. 187

460. ______ base excess
Ref. 28, p. 189

461. ______ buffer
Ref. 28, p. 189

462. ______ H_2CO_3
Ref. 28, p. 189

463. ______ pH
Ref. 28, p. 194

464. ______ standard bicarbonate
Ref. 28, p. 195

465. ______ torr
Ref. 28, p. 195

466. ______ oxygen content
Ref. 28, p. 194

467. ______ lactic acid
Ref. 28, p. 192

468. ______ bicarbonate ion
Ref. 28, p. 189

469. ______ cation
Ref. 28, p. 190

Column B

a. same as mm Hg
b. a logarithmic scale denoting hydrogen ion concentration
c. the product of anaerobic metabolic pathways
d. a substance capable of donating a hydrogen ion
e. HCO_3
f. total oxygen in blood
g. the measurement of plasma bicarbonate at a P_{CO_2} of 40 mm Hg
h. a substance that will accept hydrogen ions
i. a negatively charged ion
j. abnormal acidity of the blood
k. abnormal alkalinity of the blood
l. the number of milliequivalents per liter of bicarbonate above the normal base buffer level
m. a substance capable of neutralizing both acids and bases without changing the pH
n. the major blood acid
o. a positively charged ion

470. The ratio of H_2CO_3 to HCO_3^- is normally:
a. 5:1
b. 20:1
c. 1:10
d. 1:20
e. 10:1 *Ref. 28, p. 48*

471. A substance which by its presence in a solution is capable of minimizing changes in pH caused by the addition of acids or bases is:
a. an ion
b. a catalyst
c. a buffer
d. an enzyme
e. a regulator *Ref. 2, p. 110*

472. In an infant or neonate in a distressed or shocked state, which of the following is not a suitable area for blood gas analysis?
a. radial artery
b. temporal artery
c. capillary
d. umbilical artery
e. none of these *Ref. 2, p. 160*

473. Capillary blood gases are useful because:
a. only a small quantity of blood is needed
b. infant arteries are difficult to enter
c. the sample area can be squeezed
d. all of these
e. a and b *Ref. 78, p. 76*

474. In an infant or neonate, blood is most often obtained from what areas for capillary blood gas analysis?
a. hand
b. ear
c. finger
d. foot
e. a and d *Ref. 79, p. 212*

475. Arterial blood or arterialized capillary blood should not be collected in a:
a. glass syringe
b. plastic syringe
c. capillary tube
d. unmodified vacutainer
e. b and d *Refs. 80, p. 610; 81, p. 518*

476. In order to obtain an arterialized capillary blood sample, the clinician should:
a. warm the area
b. dilate the area by coldness
c. squeeze the area following puncture
d. avoid warming or cooling the area
e. run the sample immediately

Ref. 2, pp. 115, 116

477. Squeezing an infant's heel after puncture for capillary blood may produce:
a. coagulation
b. hemodilution
c. alkalosis
d. CO_2 retention
e. none of these *Ref. 33, p. 242*

478. In a newborn infant, arterial blood samples are not obtainable from the:
a. umbilical artery
b. radial artery
c. brachial artery
d. femoral artery
e. temporal artery *Ref. 2, p. 116*

479. After the newborn period, the _____ artery is not readily available.
a. radial
b. brachial
c. temporal
d. umbilical
e. femoral *Ref. 25, p. 155*

480. The recommended artery for blood gas sampling in children is:

a. brachial
b. radial
c. ulnar
d. femoral
e. all of these *Ref. 20, p. 160*

481. When drawing arterial blood gases, heparin is used in the syringe to:

a. provide a seal
b. displace air from the syringe and needle
c. prevent clotting
d. all of these
e. a and c *Ref. 25, p. 155*

482. Which of the following anticoagulants is suitable for use in collection of blood gas samples?

a. citrate
b. oxalate
c. sodium heparin
d. EDTA
e. potassium heparin *Ref. 2, p. 116*

483. 0.15 ml of 1000 units/ml of heparin will:

a. dissolve a clot in the blood gas analyzer
b. keep 100 ml of blood from clotting for 6 hours
c. keep 10 ml of blood from clotting for 25 minutes
d. fill the deadspace of a 5 ml-syringe
e. none of these *Ref. 28, p. 167*

484. Which of the following substances are suitable for lubrication of blood gas syringes?

a. EDTA
b. oxalate
c. ammonium heparin
d. sodium heparin
e. all are suitable *Ref. 28, p. 167*

485. Umbilical vessel catheterization is useful for:

a. administration of blood
b. withdrawing arterial blood for analysis

c. administration of bicarbonate
d. administration of electrolytes
e. all of these *Ref. 35, p. 211*

486. When ordering routine arterial blood gas analysis, the physician does not receive information concerning:
a. pH
b. Pa_{O_2}
c. Pa_{CO_2}
d. Hb
e. % saturation *Ref. 78, p. 76*

487. Every blood gas sample should be interpreted with which of the following information in mind?
a. is the patient receiving oxygen therapy
b. has the patient been suctioned recently
c. is the patient hypothermic or hyperthermic
d. all of these
e. a and b *Ref. 78, p. 76*

488. All blood gas measurements are made at:
a. STP
b. ATPS
c. BTPS
d. PSIG
e. PSIA *Ref. 28, p. 11*

489. Which substance is found in the Severinghaus electrode?
a. sodium
b. chloride
c. ammonium
d. bicarbonate
e. potassium *Ref. 82, p. 15*

490. The Severinghaus electrode measures:
a. oxygen
b. carbon dioxide
c. CO_2 content
d. base excess
e. O_2 saturation *Ref. 82, p. 15*

491. The Siggard-Andersen nomogram does not plot:
a. PCO_2
b. pH
c. B.E.
d. O_2 saturation
e. HCO_3 *Ref. 83, p. 39*

492. Which statement is *not* true of arterial punctures?
a. the blood must be heparinized
b. a glass or plastic syringe may be used
c. the radial or brachial artery may be used
d. the skin area should be cleansed with alcohol
e. with the newer techniques no pressure need be applied to the wound *Ref. 28, p. 170*

493. Which of the following is calculated rather than directly measured in the blood gas laboratory?
a. pH
b. PCO_2
c. PO_2
d. base excess
e. none of these *Ref. 2, p. 117*

494. The laboratory measurement of pH, Pa_{CO_2}, Pa_{O_2}, SO_2 and Hb makes which of these calculations possible?
a. physiologic shunt
b. base excess
c. deadspace-tidal volume ratio
d. alveolar-arterial oxygen tension difference
e. arterial-venous oxygen content difference
Ref. 28, p. 9

495. If the blood gas values from the laboratory do not correlate with the patient's condition, the clinician should check:
a. the calibration of the blood gas machine
b. the competency of the operator
c. to be sure the sample was kept aerobic
d. all of these
e. a and b *Ref. 78, p. 76*

496. The physiologic assessment of the adequacy of ventilation is reflected in the measurement of:

a. Pa_{CO_2}
b. Pa_{O_2}
c. pH
d. SO_2
e. HCO_3 *Ref. 28, p. 29*

497. The basic objection to using venous blood for monitoring is:

a. it is usually drawn from an extremity
b. it reflects local metabolic activity
c. repeated punctures carry a risk of damage to the vessel
d. it must be arterialized
e. a tourniquet must be used *Ref. 26, p. 400*

498. Which of these blood gases are closest to being normal for a neonate?

a. pH 7.35–7.45, PO_2 95–100 mm Hg, PCO_2 45–55 mm Hg
b. pH 7.35–7.40, PO_2 70–90 mm Hg, PCO_2 35–40 mm Hg
c. pH 7.2–7.25, PO_2 95–100 mm Hg, PCO_2 35–45 mm Hg
d. pH 7.2–7.25, PO_2 80 mm Hg, PCO_2 30–35 mm Hg
e. all of these are incorrect because a neonatal PO_2 is measured in torr *Ref. 57, p. 124*

499. Pa_{O_2} means:

a. partial pressure of oxygen in the airways
b. partial pressure of oxygen in the alveolar gas
c. partial pressure of oxygen in the arterial blood
d. any of these
e. none of these *Ref. 28, p. 12*

500. Pa_{CO_2} means:

a. partial pressure of arterial carbon dioxide
b. partial pressure of alveolar carbon dioxide
c. partial pressure of airway carbon dioxide
d. any of these
e. none of these *Ref. 28, p. 12*

501. Normal Pa_{O_2} in infants at birth is:
a. 30–50 mm Hg
b. 40–60 mm Hg
c. 50–70 mm Hg
d. 70–90 mm Hg
e. 90–100 mm Hg *Ref. 28, p. 91*

502. Normal Pa_{CO_2} in infants at birth is:
a. 25 mm Hg
b. 30 mm Hg
c. 34 mm Hg
d. 40 mm Hg
e. 45 mm Hg *Ref. 36, p. 3*

503. The normal Pa_{CO_2} for the first 2 years of life is:
a. 20 mm Hg
b. 30 mm Hg
c. 34 mm Hg
d. 40 mm Hg
e. 45 mm Hg *Ref. 36, p. 3*

504. An increase in the arterial P_{CO_2} will:
a. cause a rise in the pH of the blood
b. cause a fall in the pH of the blood
c. not affect the pH of the blood
d. cause a fall in the pH of the blood only in the presence of oxygen lack
e. cause hypoxemia *Ref. 28, p. 57*

505. Normal base excess at birth is:
a. zero
b. −3 mEq/L
c. −6 mEq/L
d. +5 mEq/L
e. (−6) to (+6) mEq/L *Ref. 36, p. 5*

506. A base deficit of a position value greater than −6 indicates:
a. a nonvolatile acid excess
b. a nonvolatile acid deficit
c. a 20:1 ratio in HCO_3 and CO_2

d. a normal patient's base excess
e. hyperventilation *Ref. 28, p. 55*

507. Base excess is considered an indication of:
a. the oxygen concentration in the blood
b. pulmonary disorders
c. metabolic or nonpulmonary disorders
d. HCO_3 / CO_2 content
e. H_2CO_3 / HCO_3 *Ref. 28, p. 55*

Match the following acid-base disorders with their abnormalities:

a. respiratory acidosis
b. respiratory alkalosis
c. metabolic acidosis
d. metabolic alkalosis

		B.E.	HCO_3	P_{CO_2}	pH
508.	______	−15	10.4	25	7.25
509.	______	+11	34.5	40	7.55
510.	______	+10	36.0	60	7.40
511.	______	−5	15.0	20	7.50

Ref. 76, p. 147

512. An increase in the arterial carbon dioxide tension will result in:
a. increased tidal volume
b. decreased tidal volume
c. increased tidal volume and respiratory rate
d. decrease in respiratory rate and an increase in tidal volume
e. none of these *Ref. 26, p. 120*

513. An infant is breathing 40% oxygen on a mechanical ventilator. The blood gas values are: pH 7.26, Pa_{CO_2} 60, Pa_{O_2} 60. The patient's condition is best referred to as:
a. respiratory alkalosis
b. respiratory acidosis
c. metabolic alkalosis
d. metabolic acidosis
e. alveolar hyperventilation *Ref. 28, p. 57*

514. A comatose child arrives at the emergency room of a hospital. His respirations are both rapid and shallow. Arterial puncture is performed and the blood gases are measured. If the Pa_{CO_2} is 75 mm Hg and the pH is 7.25, the correct description for this condition is which of the following?

a. respiratory acidosis
b. respiratory alkalosis
c. metabolic acidosis
d. metabolic alkalosis
e. none of these *Ref. 28, p. 57*

515. Metabolic acidosis may be caused by:

a. overexcitability of the nervous system
b. retention of CO_2
c. hyperventilation
d. absorption of excessive amounts of $NaHCO_3$
e. lactic acid in extracellular fluid *Ref. 11, p. 438*

516. Metabolic alkalosis may be caused by:

a. ingestion of sodium bicarbonate
b. a loss of alkali
c. excessive vomiting of gastric contents
d. a and c
e. b and c *Ref. 11, p. 438*

517. Severe diarrhea is one of the most frequent causes of:

a. respiratory acidosis
b. respiratory alkalosis
c. metabolic acidosis
d. metabolic alkalosis
e. none of these *Ref. 11, p. 438*

518. The major effect of alkalosis on the body is overexcitability of the nervous system. This may result in:

a. tetany
b. hypoxemia
c. uremia
d. hypercapnia
e. all of these *Ref. 11, p. 439*

519. The most common neonatal clinical entities in which respiratory acidosis occurs are:
a. perinatal asphyxia
b. choanal atresia
c. hyaline membrane disease
d. a and b
e. a and c *Ref. 2, p. 113*

520. By using the Henderson-Hasselbalch equation, the clinician can calculate:
a. PO_2
b. B.E.
c. pH
d. % saturation
e. Hb *Ref. 11, p. 429*

521. The Henderson-Hasselbalch equation interrelates which of the following?
a. PO_2, PCO_2, HCO_3^-
b. pH, PCO_2, HCO_3^-
c. HCO_3, PO_2, pH
d. PCO_2, HCO_3^-, Cl^-
e. PO_2, PCO_2, pH *Ref. 28, p. 57*

522. Which of the following is a constant in the Henderson-Hasselbalch equation as applied to the $H_2CO_3/NaHCO_3$ buffer system?
a. pH
b. pK
c. HCO_3
d. H_2CO_3
e. none of these *Ref. 76, p. 25*

523. Which of the following are measurements of gases?
a. pH, PO_2, PCO_2
b. PO_2, O_2 saturation, HCO_3^-
c. HCO_3^-, PCO_2, O_2 saturation
d. PO_2, PCO_2, O_2 saturation
e. pH, B.E., PO_2 *Ref. 28, p. 7*

524. (HCO_3^-) + (dissolved CO_2 gas) + (H_2CO_3) equals:
a. Pa_{CO_2}
b. PA_{CO_2}
c. total CO_2 content
d. dissolved CO_2
e. none of these *Ref. 26, p. 115*

525. In which acid-base disorder is there a primary retention of carbon dioxide?
a. respiratory acidosis
b. metabolic acidosis
c. respiratory alkalosis
d. metabolic alkalosis
e. none of these *Ref. 83, p. 31*

526. The arterial blood gas tensions of a spontaneously breathing infant at sea level are: pH 7.30, P_{CO_2} 50, P_{O_2} 40. These values are consistent with which of the following conditions?
a. alveolar hypoventilation
b. alveolar hyperventilation
c. metabolic acidosis
d. venous admixture
e. histotoxic hypoxia *Ref. 26, p. 119*

527. As a clinician, you have been asked how to correct a condition in a neonate in which the blood gas tensions are: Pa_{O_2} 40 mm Hg, Pa_{CO_2} 60 mm Hg, pH 7.40. Which of the following would you recommend first?
a. hyberbaric oxygen
b. hood therapy
c. 100% oxygen by incubator
d. mechanical ventilation
e. none of these *Ref. 84, pp. 194–195*

528. A patient with respiratory acidosis will manifest hypoventilation by:
a. a small tidal volume
b. tachypnea
c. bradypnea
d. a and b
e. a and c *Ref. 26, p. 121*

529. The formula bicarbonate mEq needed = body weight (kg) × 0.3 × B.E. is used to correct:

a. respiratory acidosis
b. metabolic acidosis
c. respiratory alkalosis
d. metabolic alkalosis
e. none of these *Ref. 83, p. 52*

Match the following acid-base disturbances with the possible etiology:

530. ______ vomiting *Ref. 11, p. 438*
531. ______ tetany *Ref. 60, p. 187*
532. ______ mechanical hypoventilation *Ref. 26, p. 119*
533. ______ mechanical hyperventilation *Ref. 26, p. 121*
534. ______ severe diarrhea *Ref. 11, p. 438*
535. ______ ingestion of $NaHCO_3$ *Ref. 11, p. 438*
536. ______ Diamox therapy *Ref. 85, p. 62*
537. ______ lactic acidosis *Ref. 11, p. 438*
538. ______ head trauma *Ref. 26, p. 119*
539. ______ diabetic ketoacidosis *Ref. 40, p. 639*
540. ______ treatment with Diamox *Ref. 26, p. 122*
541. ______ salicylate poisoning *Ref. 40, p. 1188*

a. respiratory acidosis
b. respiratory alkalosis
c. metabolic acidosis
d. metabolic alkalosis

542. The kidneys regulate hydrogen ion concentration by increasing or decreasing ______ reabsorption or excretion.
a. chloride
b. sodium
c. bicarbonate
d. potassium
e. ammonium *Ref. 11, p. 433*

543. The most important urine buffer is:
a. phosphate
b. bicarbonate
c. ammonium
d. sodium
e. potassium *Ref. 28, p. 53*

544. For the bicarbonate buffer system the pK is:
a. 6.1
b. 6.8
c. 7.0
d. 7.4
e. 7.8 *Ref. 11, p 429*

545. The plasma bicarbonate ion concentration is under the primary control of the:
a. respiratory system
b. renal system
c. muscle system
d. skeletal system
e. nervous system *Ref. 28, p. 50*

546. A drug is listed in the United States Pharmacopeia (U.S.P.) after:
a. its safety has been demonstrated in animals
b. its safety has been demonstrated in humans
c. it has been shown to be both reasonably safe and effective in humans and has become widely used
d. it meets the standards of U.S.P.
e. none of these *Ref. 85, p. xiv*

547. According to medical terminology, a drug can be defined as:
a. a substance which causes destruction of cells

b. a chemical agent which affects living protoplasm
c. a chemical substance that is readily absorbed from the gastrointestinal tract
d. a chemical agent used in the treatment, prevention or diagnosis of a disease
e. none of these *Ref. 1, p. 378*

In column A are listed various preparations. In column B are found their definitions. Match column A with column B.

Column A

548. ______ tablet
549. ______ capsule
550. ______ lozenge
551. ______ ampule
552. ______ solution
553. ______ elixir
554. ______ syrup
555. ______ multiple-dose vial
556. ______ tincture
557. ______ suppository

Column B

a. flavored tablets which dissolve slowly when held in the mouth
b. an alcoholic extract of a drug
c. contains the drug in a concentrated sugar solution
d. the most common preparation for oral use
e. a drug container made of gelatin that will disintegrate in water
f. a glass container in which solutions of drugs are protected until administered
g. rubber-stoppered containers from which several doses can be withdrawn
h. a sweet, aromatic, dilute alcoholic solution of a drug
i. an aqueous preparation of a drug
j. a drug inserted into the vagina or rectum

Ref. 86, p. 21

In column A are listed some pharmacological abbreviations used daily in medicine. Column B gives the definition for which the abbreviation is used. Match column A with B.

Column A	Column B
558. ______ āā	a. write on label
559. ______ a.c.	b. thrice each day
560. ______ ad lib.	c. without
561. ______ b.i.d.	d. grain
562. ______ c̄	e. hour
563. ______ gtt.	f. 4 times each day
564. ______ gm	g. one half
565. ______ gr.	h. a quantity sufficient to make
566. ______ h.	i. milligram
567. ______ h.s.	j. every
568. ______ mcg	k. after meals
569. ______ mg	l. to be repeated
570. ______ non repetat.	m. drops
571. ______ p.c.	n. immediately
572. ______ p.r.n.	o. of each
573. ______ q.	p. twice each day
574. ______ q.i.d.	q. gram
575. ______ q.s. ad	r. at bedtime
576. ______ Rep.	s. as the need arises
577. ______ s̄	t. before meals
578. ______ Sig.	u. not to be repeated
579. ______ s̄s̄.	v. microgram
580. ______ stat.	w. with
581. ______ t.i.d.	x. freely

Ref. 86, pp. 23–24

582. If a child is to receive 5 mg p.c. and h.s. of Drug X by inhalation, at which times during the day would the drug be administered?

a. after meals
b. before arising
c. after bedtime and before arising
d. after meals and at bedtime
e. before meals and after bedtime

Ref. 86, pp. 23–24

583. The safest and most economical method of administering the majority of drugs is:

a. orally
b. intramuscularly
c. intravenously
d. subcutaneously
e. rectally *Ref. 86, p. 18*

584. A desirable or undesirable effect of a drug other than the therapeutic one for which the drug was given is defined as:

a. toxicity
b. allergic reaction
c. side-effect
d. drug abuse
e. synergistic effect *Ref. 87, p. 6*

585. The most important factor influencing the safety and effectiveness of a drug in a clinicial situation is:

a. hypersensitivity
b. tolerance
c. drug allergy
d. competence of the prescriber
e. biological variation *Ref. 86, p. 24*

586. If a patient develops tolerance to a drug, it means he:

a. built up a sensitivity to the drug
b. obtained the maximum response of the drug
c. has no therapeutic need for the drug
d. needs an increasing dosage to maintain the initial effect
e. had an unexpected side-effect *Ref. 86, p. 20*

587. All of the following are advantages of intravenous administration of a drug except:

a. can give highly irritating substances
b. can titrate for exact response
c. can decrease the dose once given
d. can administer drug over a long period of time
e. can give an accurate dose for a particular response *Ref. 86, p. 19*

588. Which of the following may depress respiration?

a. narcotics
b. barbituates
c. diuretics
d. all of these
e. a and b *Ref. 86, pp. 202, 240*

589. Alpha receptors are responsible for all of the following except:

a. vasoconstriction
b. iris dilation
c. bronchial relaxation
d. cardioacceleration
e. none of these *Ref. 11, p. 698*

590. Which of the following is the excitatory receptor of the adrenergic branch of the autonomic nervous system?

a. alpha receptor
b. $beta_1$ receptor
c. $beta_2$ receptor
d. a and b
e. a and c *Ref. 86, p. 73*

591. Most commonly used bronchodilators are:

a. parasympathomimetic
b. analeptic
c. cholinergic
d. analgesic
e. none of these *Ref. 26, p. 189*

592. Which one is not a sympathomimetic amine?

a. Emivan
b. isoproterenol
c. racemic epinephrine
d. cyclopentamine hydrochloride
e. phenylephrine hydrochloride *Ref. 85, p. 104*

593. An example of a drug which is not a bronchodilator is:

a. ephedrine
b. aminophylline
c. isoproterenol
d. Bronkosol

e. none of these *Ref. 85, pp. 96, 98, 100, 121*

594. Which of the following drugs has no bronchodilator effect?

a. Isuprel
b. Bronkosol
c. Mucomyst
d. Dornavac
e. c and d *Ref. 85, pp. 74–75*

595. All of the following agents can be used as bronchodilators except:

a. aminophylline
b. epinephrine
c. norepinephrine
d. isoetharine
e. isoproterenol *Ref. 87, p. 64*

596. Bronchodilators *cannot* be administered via:

a. IPPB
b. aerosol
c. hand nebulizer
d. micronebulizer
e. cascade humidifier *Ref. 85, p. 98*

597. An increase in pulse rate during IPPB administration of a bronchodilator indicates:

a. systemic absorption of the drug
b. cardiac disease
c. respiratory disease
d. side-effects of the drug
e. the patient is not tolerating the drug

Ref. 48, pp. 192–93

598. Sympathomimetic drugs are:

a. direct stimulants of alpha and beta receptors
b. indirect and direct stimulants of alpha and beta receptors
c. direct stimulants of alpha receptors only
d. direct stimulants of beta receptors only
e. all of these *Ref. 85, p. 93*

599. Which of the following drugs is *not* an alpha stimulator?
a. Bronkosol
b. Isuprel
c. Decadron
d. aminophylline
e. a and b *Ref. 85, pp. 98, 100*

600. Which of the following drugs contains phenylephrine hydrochloride?
a. Bronkosol
b. Isuprel
c. Neo-Synephrine
d. all of these
e. a and c *Ref. 85, p. 105*

601. Bronkosol has primarily:
a. $beta_2$ stimulation only
b. alpha stimulation only
c. alpha and $beta_1$ stimulation
d. $beta_1$ and $beta_2$ stimulation
e. none of these *Ref. 85, p. 98*

602. Bronkosol may be used for:
a. bronchial asthma
b. bronchospasms
c. emphysema
d. chronic bronchitis
e. all of these *Ref. 85, p. 98*

603. Bronkosol-2 contains what other ingredient?
a. isoetharine hydrochloride
b. Dilabron
c. phenylephrine hydrochloride
d. thenyldiamine hydrochloride
e. water *Ref. 85, p. 98*

604. What specific action does isoetharine hydrochloride in Bronkosol have?
a. bronchodilation
b. antifoaming
c. anti-inflammatory
d. stimulant

e. decongestant *Ref. 85, p. 98*

605. The peak response time of isoetharine is:

a. 5 minutes
b. 10–15 minutes
c. 30 minutes
d. 60 minutes
e. immediately *Ref. 88*

606. Bronkosol can be administered by which of these methods?

a. intramuscular
b. intravenous
c. inhalation
d. rectal suppository
e. all of these *Ref. 85, p. 98*

607. Which of the following is usually a contraindication for the use of Bronkosol?

a. bronchitis
b. hypersensitivity to any ingredient
c. asthma
d. all of these
e. a and b *Ref. 85, p. 98*

608. Isuprel is a:

a. peripheral vasoconstrictor
b. sympathomimetic amine
c. cardiac inhibitor
d. all of these
e. a and b *Ref. 85, pp. 93–100*

609. Isuprel contains:

a. cyclopentamine
b. isoetharine
c. thenyldiamine
d. sodium citrate
e. isoproterenol sulfate *Ref. 71, p. 244*

610. Possible side-effects of Isuprel can be:
a. headache
b. nausea
c. palpitation
d. tachycardia
e. all of these *Ref. 85, p. 100*

611. The 1:100 preparation of isoproterenol hydrochloride contains:
a. phenylephrine hydrochloride
b. glycerin
c. saccharin
d. thenyldiamine hydrochloride
e. cyclopentamine hydrochloride *Ref. 71, p. 244*

612. The 1:200 preparation of isoproterenol hydrochloride contains:
a. phenylephrine hydrochloride
b. glycerin
c. saccharin
d. thenyldiamine hydrochloride
e. cyclopentamine hydrochloride *Ref. 71, p. 244*

613. Isoproterenol should not be used concurrently with:
a. sympathomimetic amines
b. racemic epinephrine
c. isoetharine
d. a and c
e. none of these *Ref. 85, p. 100*

614. The physician has ordered 5 ml of a 1:100 solution of isoproterenol p.r.n. by inhalation. How much Isuprel would the patient receive over a 24-hour period?
a. 5 ml
b. 5 mg
c. 10 mg
d. 10 ml
e. cannot be determined *Ref. 85, pp. 127–133*

615. Adverse reactions (side-effects) of Isuprel and Bronkosol as bronchodilators might include all of the following except:
a. tachycardia
b. nervousness
c. vomiting
d. palpitation
e. sedation *Ref. 85, p. 100*

616. Cromolyn sodium is the generic name for:
a. Intal
b. Aarane
c. isoetharine
d. a and b
e. a and c *Ref. 85, p. 48*

617. Cromolyn sodium has a role in:
a. treatment of acute asthmatic attack
b. treatment of emphysema
c. management of patients with perennial asthma
d. all of these
e. a and b *Ref. 85, p. 48*

618. Cromolyn sodium is administered via:
a. intravenous route
b. inhalation
c. intramuscular injection
d. capsule
e. tablet *Ref. 85, p. 48*

619. Epinephrine is a:
a. bronchodilator and vasodilator
b. bronchoconstrictor and vasoconstrictor
c. bronchodilator-vasoconstrictor
d. bronchoconstrictor-vasodilator
e. bronchodilator only *Ref. 85, p. 97*

620. Epinephrine is:
a. a cardiac stimulant
b. another name for adrenaline
c. a substance in Bronkosol
d. all of these
e. a and b *Ref. 85, p. 97*

621. Epinephrine acts on which of the following?

a. alpha receptors
b. $beta_1$ receptors
c. $beta_2$ receptors
d. all of these
e. a and c *Ref. 85, p. 97*

622. Another name for epinephrine is:

a. Intal
b. Aarane
c. theophylline
d. adrenaline
e. isoetharine *Ref. 85, p. 97*

623. Mucomyst contains:

a. 20% acetylcysteine
b. 30% acetylcysteine
c. 40% acetylcysteine
d. 50% acetylcysteine
e. 60% acetylcysteine *Ref. 85, p. 74*

624. In what concentration is Mucomyst available?

a. 10%
b. 20%
c. 30%
d. a and b
e. b and c *Ref. 85, p. 74*

625. Which drug will likely cause bronchospasm in patients with asthma?

a. Mucomyst
b. Aerosporin
c. Dornavac
d. ethyl alcohol
e. Aarane *Ref. 85, p. 74*

626. A drug with a rotten-egg odor is:

a. Intal
b. Aarane
c. Mucomyst
d. Bronkosol
e. Dornavac *Ref. 26, p. 200*

627. A drug which is often instilled into endotracheal tubes to facilitate liquefaction is:
a. Dornavac
b. NaCl
c. Mucomyst
d. Bronkosol
e. distilled water *Ref. 26, p. 200*

628. Pancreatic dornase is a:
a. detergent
b. bronchodilator
c. enzyme
d. antifoaming agent
e. steroid *Ref. 85, p. 75*

629. The trade name for pancreatic dornase is:
a. Bronkosol
b. Dornavac
c. Intal
d. Aarane
e. Nebuprel *Ref. 85, p. 75*

630. Pancreatic dornase is derived from:
a. protein of the beef pancreas
b. the pancreas of a fetal pig
c. DNA
d. dornase
e. beef lung *Ref. 85, p. 75*

631. DNA protein in mucus is:
a. usually present
b. denatured by Dornavac
c. a cause of viscosity
d. all of these
e. none of these *Ref. 12, p. 36*

632. Clinically, Dornavac is not indicated in:
a. pulmonary abscess
b. bronchiectasis
c. bronchitis
d. cystic fibrosis
e. conditions with purulent sputum
Ref. 26, p. 203

633. A drug which often causes a burning sensation in the mouth following an IPPB treatment is:
a. ethyl alcohol
b. Mucomyst
c. Dornavac
d. Decadron
e. Vaponefrin *Ref. 26, p. 203*

634. A decongestant is a type of drug that:
a. provides mucolytic properties
b. acts as a vasodilator
c. has bronchodilating effects
d. constricts arterioles and small arteries
e. constricts venules and small veins
Ref. 26, p. 188

635. Ethyl alcohol is used in pulmonary edema:
a. for its bacteriostatic effects
b. for nebulization
c. to lower the surface tension of froth
d. to eliminate the diffusion barrier
e. none of these *Ref. 26, p. 201*

636. A drug which is useful in treating *Pseudomonas aeruginosa* infections is:
a. Lasix
b. nitrogylcerin
c. Kantrex
d. Aerosporin
e. Bicillin *Ref. 85, p. 19*

637. Neostigmine is:
a. parasympatholytic
b. an alpha stimulant
c. sympathomimetic
d. an acetylcholinesterase inhibitor
e. a and c *Ref. 85, p. 25*

638. Neo-Synephrine is used primarily:
a. as a nasal decongestant
b. as an anti-inflammatory agent
c. as a topical agent

d. to cause diuresis
e. as an antifoaming agent *Ref. 85, p. 104*

639. The chemical name for aminophylline is:
a. theophylline ethylenediamine
b. caffeine sulfate
d. theobromine sulfide
d. xanthine hydrochloride
e. Aerosporin *Ref. 85, p. 121*

640. The side-effects of aminophylline administration include all of the following except:
a. nausea
b. palpitation
c. headache
d. tachycardia
e. an increase in blood pressure *Ref. 85, p. 121*

641. Generally speaking, a steroid's action is that of:
a. reducing surface tension
b. reducing the viscosity of purulent mucus
c. being anti-inflammatory
d. providing relief of severe bronchospasm
e. cardioregulation *Ref. 85, p. 1*

642. Excessive administration of $NaHCO_3$ can result in:
a. alkalosis
b. hypocalcemia
c. hypokalemia
d. hypernatremia
e. all of these *Ref. 33, p. 30*

643. A drug which is used to abolish the sensation of pain is called:
a. a diuretic
b. an analgesic
c. an aseptic
d. an analeptic
e. an anesthetic *Ref. 1, p. 57*

644. Nausea, stomatitis and bronchospasm are possible side-effects of:
a. isoetharine
b. cromolyn sodium
c. acetylcysteine
d. pancreatic dornase
e. Vaponefrin *Ref. 85, p. 74*

645. If respiratory depression of the newborn infant is suspected as the result of maternal overdose of CNS depressants, a drug which can be given to the infant is:
a. Lorfan
b. levallorphan tartrate
c. Nalline
d. all of these
e. a and b *Ref. 89, p. 186*

646. Morphine sulfate is:
a. a sedative
b. an analgesic
c. a tranquilizer
d. a barbiturate
e. an antibiotic *Ref. 85, p. 81*

647. The standard I.V. solution used to replace simple water loss in a patient is:
a. 5% dextrose in water
b. physiological saline
c. 5% sodium bicarbonate
d. sterile distilled water
e. Ringer's lactate *Ref. 90, p. 87*

648. All of the following are diuretics except:
a. Diamox
b. Lasix
c. Xylocaine
d. Edecrin
e. xanthine *Ref. 85, pp. 61–66*

649. Neuromuscular blocking agents include all of the following except:
a. succinylcholine chloride

b. curare
c. Anectine
d. mephenesin
e. none of these *Ref. 85, pp. 40–42*

650. A sympathomimetic used in cases of complete atrial-ventricular block is:
a. Bronkosol
b. digitalis
c. Pronestyl
d. quinidine
e. isoproterenol *Ref. 85, p. 50*

651. The slowest- and longest-acting cardiac glycoside is:
a. digoxin
b. nitroglycerin
c. digitoxin
d. ouabain
e. quinidine *Ref. 85, p. 57*

652. All of the following are effects of histamine except:
a. constricts veins
b. increases capillary permeability
c. vasodilates arterioles
d. all of these
e. a and c *Ref. 11, p. 296*

653. All of the following are used as skeletal muscle relaxants except:
a. succinylcholine chloride
b. neostigmine
c. *d*-tubocurarine
d. Anectine
e. none of these *Ref. 85, p. 25*

654. Which of the following dosages quantitatively possesses the most drug?
a. 1:100
b. 1:200
c. 1:400
d. 1:600
e. 1:1000 *Ref. 85, p. 131*

In column A several drugs are listed by their proprietary names. In column B are listed their generic names. Match columns A and B.

Column A	Column B
655. ______ Isuprel *Ref. 85, p. 100*	a. cyclopentamine
656. ______ Dornavac *Ref. 85, p. 75*	b. neomycin sulfate
657. ______ Varidase *Ref. 85, p. 76*	c. isoproterenol hydrochloride
658. ______ saline *Ref. 85, p. 90*	d. acetylcysteine
659. ______ Mucomyst *Ref. 85, p. 74*	e. streptokinase
660. ______ Aerolone *Ref. 85, p. 99*	f. pancreatic dornase
661. ______ Mycifradin *Ref. 85, p. 17*	g. 0.9% sodium chloride in water

In column A are listed several characteristics or components of drugs. In column B are listed several drugs. Match column A to Column B.

Column A	Column B
662. ______ enzymatic in action *Ref. 85, p. 75*	a. Dornavac
663. ______ antibiotic in action *Ref. 85, p. 16*	b. saline
664. ______ breaks down disulfide bonds *Ref. 85, p. 74*	c. Aerolone
665. ______ closest representative of body fluid *Ref. 85, p. 90*	d. Isuprel
666. ______ contains glycerin *Ref. 85, p. 100*	e. Mucomyst
667. ______ contains two bronchodilators *Ref. 85, p. 99*	f. ethyl alcohol
668. ______ cardiac stimulant *Ref. 85, p. 100*	g. neomycin sulfate

669. ______ antifoaming agent
Ref. 85, p. 92

670. ______ an electrolyte balancer
Ref. 85, p. 90

671. ______ contains acetylcysteine
Ref. 85, p. 74

672. When administering a bronchodilator, one should monitor:
a. pulse
b. blood pressure
c. ECG
d. number of respirations
e. temperature *Ref. 48, p. 226*

673. While drugs are being administered intravenously, the clinician should:
a. carefully monitor the rate of administration
b. closely observe the patient's reactions
c. report side-effects to the physician
d. all of these
e. a and c *Ref. 40, p. 1144*

674. A drug which is not useful in the treatment of asthma is:
a. epinephrine
b. aminophylline
c. ephedrine
d. acetylcysteine
e. Bronkosol *Ref. 40, p. 1143*

675. Which of the following methods of drug administration is not used to deliver aminophylline?
a. inhalation
b. intravenous
c. topical
d. rectal
e. none of these *Ref. 85, p. 121*

676. Which group of medications is generally administered to cystic fibrosis patients?
a. antibiotics
b. expectorants
c. bronchodilators
d. all of these
e. a and b *Ref. 40, p. 1211*

677. The drug of choice for treatment of an acute asthmatic attack is:
a. ephedrine
b. isoproterenol
c. epinephrine
d. Bronkosol
e. Intal *Ref. 91, p. 31*

678. Which of the following drugs is not used routinely in the treatment of asthma?
a. epinephrine
b. isoproterenol
c. Intal
d. aminophylline
e. Lasix *Ref. 85, pp. 48, 97, 100, 121*

679. Occasionally an infant is neurologically depressed secondary to narcotic sedation of the mother. Treatment requires administration of:
a. morphine
b. nalorphine
c. reserpine
d. atropine
e. tetracycline *Ref. 25, p. 35*

In column A are listed several commonly used drugs. In column B are their general classifications. Match column A with Column B.

Column A	Column B
680. ______ Lasix *Ref. 85, p. 66*	a. bronchodilator
	b. mucolytic
681. ______ Valium *Ref. 85, p. 109*	c. antibiotic
	d. antifoaming agent

682. ______ isoetharine
Ref. 85, p. 98
683. ______ quinidine
Ref. 85, p. 55
684. ______ Aarane
Ref. 85, p. 48
685. ______ morphine
Ref. 85, p. 81
686. ______ Keflin
Ref. 85, p. 10
687. ______ ethyl alcohol
Ref. 85, p. 92
688. ______ acetylcysteine
Ref. 85, p. 74
689. ______ Xylocaine
Ref. 85, p. 52

e. anesthetic
f. bronchial asthma inhibitor
g. antiarrhythmic
h. diuretic
i. analgesic
j. sedative

SECTION 4

Cardiopulmonary Diseases

For each of these questions select the *one* most appropriate answer.

690. High risk infants include:
a. infants born to diabetic mothers
b. infants born to mothers who have bled during the third trimester
c. infants born to Rh-negative mothers
d. infants born to mothers who are addicts
e. all of these *Ref. 33, p. 67*

691. Noisy breathing which usually occurs during inspiration and is commonly associated with upper airway obstruction is called:
a. apnea
b. periodic respiration
c. grunting
d. stridor
e. retractions *Ref. 33, p. 105*

692. Grunting is considered abnormal if it persists longer than the first:
a. 30 minutes of life
b. 1 hour of life
c. 8 hours of life
d. day of life
e. all of these *Ref. 33, p. 105*

693. In which of these diseases is grunting typical in the newborn?
a. asthma
b. bronchiolitis
c. disseminated bronchopneumonia
d. RDS
e. all of these *Ref. 39, p. 311*

694. Apnea is:
a. shortness of breath
b. absence of respiration
c. periodic breathing
d. low frequency, but normal depth, breathing
e. none of these *Ref. 1, p. 90*

695. Complete apnea usually lasts for:
a. 5 seconds
b. 5–10 seconds
c. more than 30 seconds
d. 2–3 minutes
e. 1–5 minutes *Ref. 33, p. 105*

696. Apnea is associated with:
a. cyanosis
b. a decrease in heart rate
c. an increase in pH
d. a and b
e. b and c *Ref. 33, p. 105*

697. Periods of rapid respiration lasting about 20 seconds alternating with periods of cessation of breathing for 5–10 seconds is called:
a. apnea
b. periodic respiration
c. stridor
d. grunting
e. tachypnea *Ref. 33, p. 105*

698. Irregular breathing often increases during sleep in pediatric patients who have:
a. pickwickian syndrome
b. Riley-Day syndrome
c. bronchiolitis
d. choanal atresia
e. esophageal atresia *Ref. 4, p. 5*

699. The symptoms of a foreign body in the nose are:
a. local obstruction
b. discomfort
c. sneezing

d. all of these
e. a and b *Ref. 27, p. 884*

700. The most common congenital abnormality of the nasal passages is:
a. Wilson-Mikity syndrome
b. choanal atresia
c. micrognathia
d. transient tachypnea of the newborn
e. pectus excavatum *Ref. 27, p. 883*

701. Neonatal respiratory depression is often caused by:
a. maternal analgesia
b. maternal anesthesia
c. CNS dysfunction
d. aspiration of amniotic fluid
e. all of these *Ref. 63, p. 240*

702. Newborn infants may have cardiorespiratory problems because of:
a. asphyxia
b. maternal drugs
c. intrathoracic disease
d. anemia
e. all of these *Ref. 25, p. 35*

703. Which of the following disorders most often occurs in *infants* under 2 years of age?
a. emphysema
b. bronchitis
c. pneumonia
d. bronchiolitis
e. cystic fibrosis *Ref. 4, p. 80*

704. Intrauterine asphyxia would most likely cause:
a. choanal atresia
b. tetralogy of Fallot
c. asphyxia neonatorum
d. aspiration syndrome
e. ductus arteriosus *Ref. 4, p. 53*

705. Asphyxia neonatorum refers to:
a. suffocation
b. abnormal surfactant production
c. decreased arterial oxygen levels in the neonate
d. suffocation of the newborn
e. none of these *Ref. 1, p. 119*

706. Asphyxia neonatorum may be caused by:
a. intrauterine asphyxia
b. maternal anesthesia
c. maternal analgesia
d. upper airway obstruction
e. all of these *Ref. 4, p. 53*

707. Management of neonatal asphyxia does not consist of:
a. clearing of the upper airway
b. maintenance of body temperature
c. silver nitrate administration
d. artificial ventilation
e. cardiac massage *Ref. 4, p. 53*

708. Choanal atresia is:
a. a congenital malformation
b. sometimes found in newborns
c. an obstruction of the posterior nares
d. caused by membranous or bony structure obstruction
e. all of these *Ref. 2, pp. 146–47*

709. Choanal atresia:
a. may be unilateral
b. may be bilateral
c. may go unnoticed for years
d. can cause death if bilateral
e. all of these *Ref. 4, p. 61*

710. An infant with choanal atresia may ventilate well while:
a. sleeping
b. moving
c. crying
d. eating
e. resting *Ref. 92, p. 80*

711. A diagnosis of choanal atresia is confirmed by:
- a. x-ray of the mouth
- b. inability to insert an oral airway
- c. watching the infant mouth breathe
- d. nasal flaring with hypoxemia
- e. inability to pass a probe or tube through the nose *Ref. 4, p. 61*

712. A condition in which the openings of the nose into the nasopharynx are closed by a septum containing bone is:
- a. laryngeal stridor
- b. choanal atresia
- c. Wilson-Mikity syndrome
- d. transient tachypnea of the newborn
- e. micrognathia *Ref. 4, p. 60*

713. RDS babies usually:
- a. have a deficiency of pulmonary surfactant
- b. are premature
- c. have retractions
- d. demonstrate tachypnea and expiratory grunting
- e. all of these *Ref. 4, p. 56*

714. RDS should be suspected in infants:
- a. of diabetic mothers
- b. of mothers who are bleeding
- c. who are premature
- d. all of these
- e. a and c *Ref. 4, p. 48*

715. In the lungs of infants with hyaline membrane disease the:
- a. V_T is increased
- b. FRC is increased
- c. IRV is increased
- d. ERV is increased
- e. none of these *Ref. 32, p. 155*

716. The laboratory findings of RDS are:
a. hypoxemia
b. respiratory acidosis
c. metabolic acidosis
d. all of these
e. a and b *Ref. 33, p. 119*

717. Which of the following is not a classic symptom of RDS?
a. cyanosis
b. retractions
c. hyperoxemia
d. grunting
e. tachypnea *Ref. 21, p. 223*

718. Clinical estimations of the degree of respiratory failure in a newborn are based upon which of the following factors?
a. air entry, color and respiratory rate
b. nasal flaring, grunting and abdominal breathing
c. intercostal retractions and blood
d. measurement of arterial pH, base excess and Hb
e. all of these *Ref. 33, pp. 105–7*

719. A disorder which is not a common cause of respiratory failure in the newborn is:
a. birth asphyxia
b. respiratory distress syndrome
c. choanal atresia
d. pneumothorax
e. congenital heart disease *Ref. 35, p. 241*

720. What is coryza?
a. a head cold
b. an allergy
c. an increased temperature
d. a bronchial disorder
e. a cardiac disorder *Ref. 1, p. 293*

721. Which of the following factors are considerations in the prevention of retrolental fibroplasia?
a. FI_{O_2}

b. Pa_{O_2}
c. duration of oxygen administration
d. age of the infant
e. all of these *Ref. 93, p. 19*

722. The effect of oxygen on the retinal vessels is dependent upon:
a. the stage of development of the retinal vessels
b. the length of exposure to oxygen
c. the concentration of oxygen in the arterial blood
d. all of these
e. a and c *Ref. 25, p. 57*

723. Describe the sequence of events leading to retrolental fibroplasia:
a. high Pa_{O_2} → arteriolar vasoconstriction → regional ischemia → dilation of proximal vessels of the eyes → retinal detachment → blindness
b. high Pa_{O_2} → retinal destruction → ischemic injury → blindness
c. high Pa_{O_2} → ischemia of superior and inferior retinal arteries → fibrous tissue formation → blindness
d. all of these
e. none of these *Ref. 79, p. 281*

724. To try to avoid retrolental fibroplasia, which of the following modalities should be monitored frequently?
a. FI_{O_2}
b. Pa_{O_2}
c. FI_{O_2} and Pa_{O_2}
d. FI_{O_2} and hematocrit
e. Pa_{O_2}, R.B.C. level and hematocrit

Ref. 32, p. 156

725. Micrognathia is:
a. oversecretion of ADH
b. underutilization of epithelial cells in the kidney
c. underdevelopment of the lower jaw
d. a disease of white blood cells
e. a congenital heart disorder of neonates

Ref. 4, p. 60

726. Micrognathia is most commonly seen in association with:

a. choanal atresia
b. Pierre Robin syndrome
c. diaphragmatic hernia
d. lung cyst
e. congenital laryngeal stridor *Ref. 94, p. 265*

727. In micrognathia:

a. asphyxia never occurs
b. the patient should be placed in a supine position
c. oxygen therapy is useless
d. the tongue is abnormally small
e. stridor is unusual *Ref. 4, p. 60*

728. Micrognathia associated with cleft palate is called:

a. bilateral choanal atresia
b. foramen of Bochdalek
c. Pierre Robin syndrome
d. congenital laryngeal stridor
e. Wilson-Mikity syndrome *Ref. 30, p. 202*

729. An infant with Pierre Robin syndrome should be managed:

a. in a prone position
b. in a supine position
c. with the head hyperextended
d. in Trendelenburg's position
e. on his side *Ref. 41, p. 84*

730. Unpredictable episodes of respiratory obstruction near the base of the tongue describe:

a. Pierre Robin syndrome
b. choanal atresia
c. foramen of Bochdalek
d. Wilson-Mikity syndrome
e. bronchiolitis *Ref. 41, p. 84*

731. In a child, a foreign body most often lodges in the:

a. nose
b. pharynx
c. right main bronchus

d. left main bronchus
e. carina *Ref. 95, p. 1099*

732. If laryngeal obstruction occurs because of a foreign body, the treatment is:
a. a nasopharyngeal airway
b. an oropharyngeal airway
c. nasotracheal intubation
d. endotracheal intubation
e. tracheostomy *Ref. 95, p. 1099*

733. Tracheal foreign bodies may produce:
a. cyanosis
b. emphysema
c. decreased air entry
d. all of these
e. a and c *Ref. 95, p. 1099*

734. A symptom not common to foreign-body aspiration is:
a. choking
b. coughing
c. sneezing
d. gagging
e. wheezing *Ref. 95, p. 1099*

735. Aspirated foreign bodies may produce:
a. partial or complete obstruction
b. suffocation
c. hyperinflation of the involved lobe or segment
d. all of these
e. a and b *Ref. 70, p. 311*

736. Which of the following foreign bodies swells to many times its original size when inhaled?
a. coin
b. needle
c. peanut
d. safety pin
e. tack *Ref. 95, p. 1100*

737. Vegetable bronchitis is due to aspiration into the trachea or bronchi of organic foreign bodies such as:
a. beans
b. peanuts
c. leaves
d. grass
e. all of these *Ref. 95, p. 1100*

738. A syndrome of pulmonary disease following prolonged oxygen and ventilator therapy of RDS is:
a. foramen of Bochdalek
b. Pierre Robin syndrome
c. micrognathia
d. bronchopulmonary dysplasia
e. choanal atresia *Ref. 96, pp. 357–68*

739. Obstruction at the level of the tongue in an infant may be relieved by insertion of a:
a. nasopharyngeal airway
b. oropharyngeal airway
c. nasotracheal tube
d. orotracheal tube
e. tracheostomy tube *Ref. 41, p. 103*

740. Croup is:
a. another term for laryngotracheobronchitis
b. caused by parainfluenza virus types 1 and 2
c. inflammation of the larynx, trachea and bronchi
d. all of these
e. a and c *Ref. 1, p. 302*

741. What is most important about croup?
a. the infection
b. the level at which it occurs
c. the amount of exudate
d. the degree of obstruction
e. the symptoms *Ref. 97, p. 51*

742. Croup is usually characterized by:
a. inspiratory stridor
b. hoarseness
c. barking cough

d. laryngeal obstruction
e. all of these *Ref. 97, pp. 51–67*

743. Another name for acute laryngotracheobronchitis is:
a. acute obstructive subglottic largyngitis
b. cystic fibrosis
c. croup
d. laryngitis
e. a and c *Ref. 97, p. 60*

744. Another name for acute obstructive supraglottic laryngitis is:
a. croup
b. tracheitis
c. epiglottitis
d. pharyngitis
e. pectus excavatum *Ref. 97, p. 58*

745. In croup, the primary objective is to:
a. relieve cyanosis
b. eliminate acidosis
c. maintain a patent airway
d. reduce hypoxemia
e. reduce edema *Ref. 40, p. 1149*

746. In a child with croup, a tracheotomy is indicated when:
a. respiratory rate increases
b. cyanosis occurs
c. restlessness and apprehension occur with a pulse in excess of 160 per minute
d. sternal retractions are accompanied by increased use of accessory muscles
e. all of these *Ref. 97, p. 56*

747. In acute supraglottic obstruction, the most important sign of impending diaster is:
a. dysphagia
b. pooling of saliva in the pharynx
c. cherry-red epiglottis
d. the child leaning forward, mouth open
e. difficult breathing *Ref. 97, p. 53*

748. Which of the following is the most common cause of viral croup?
a. pneumococcus
b. staphylococcus
c. *Hemophilus influenzae*, type A_2
d. *Hemophilus influenzae*, type B
e. *Corynebacterium diphtheriae* *Ref. 25, p. 79*

749. In epiglottitis, the:
a. white blood cell count is decreased
b. epiglottis is red and swollen
c. patient's head should not be hyperextended
d. drug of choice is atropine
e. onset is slow *Ref. 97, p. 53*

750. Which of the following may be used to treat a child with croup or epiglottitis?
a. Cam tent
b. Universal croupette
c. ultrasonic nebulizer
d. croupette with high humidity
e. all of these *Ref. 25, p. 80*

751. Which of the following occurs in a croup patient?
a. cough and fever
b. stridor
c. laryngeal obstruction
d. red and edematous tracheal walls
e. all of these *Ref. 25, pp. 78–80*

752. If a child with epiglottitis receives oxygen by nasal catheter, a possible complication is:
a. abdominal distention
b. drying of secretions
c. intestinal rupture
d. all of these
e. a and c *Ref. 25, p. 100*

753. Which of the following methods of therapy is contraindicated in croup?
a. hot steam
b. cold steam

c. croupette
d. oxygen by mask
e. none of these *Ref. 25, p. 81*

754. Which of the following disorders are not infant or childhood disorders?
a. hyaline membrane disease
b. bronchial asthma
c. cystic fibrosis
d. croup
e. sarcoidosis *Ref. 4, pp. 56, 79, 81, 85*

755. Bronchiolitis is:
a. another name for croup
b. a viral illness of infants
c. often treated with oxygen by mask
d. an upper airway obstruction
e. a disease of older children *Ref. 25, p. 84*

756. The clinical manifestations of bronchiolitis are:
a. wheezing
b. dyspnea
c. sternal retractions
d. cough
e. all of these *Ref. 40, p. 1147*

757. Occasionally infants are born with a sternal disorder called funnel chest. The technical name for this is:
a. flail chest
b. pectus excavatum
c. bronchial asthma
d. Riley-Day syndrome
e. kyphoscoliosis *Ref. 4, p. 81*

758. Which of the following disorders is not a respiratory emergency in the newborn?
a. asphyxia neonatorum
b. meconium aspiration
c. congenital disphragmatic hernia
d. Wilson-Mikity syndrome
e. bilateral choanal atresia *Ref. 4, pp. 53–62*

759. During the transition from fetal to adult circulation, right-to-left shunts occur where?
a. the foramen ovale
b. the ductus arteriosus
c. intrapulmonary shunts
d. ductus venosus
e. all of these except d *Ref. 4, p. 24*

760. The purpose of fluid therapy in the infant with respiratory distress is:
a. maintenance of hydration
b. provision of calories
c. prevention of hypoglycemia
d. correction of acidosis
e. all of these *Ref. 92, pp. 86–87*

761. A severe attack of asthma which has continued for more than 24 hours is termed:
a. croup
b. bronchitis
c. status asthmaticus
d. bronchiolitis
e. respiratory failure *Ref. 98, p. 418*

762. Asthma is not clinically manifested by:
a. breathlessness
b. eupnea
c. wheezing
d. dyspnea
e. cough *Ref. 98, p. 404*

763. The etiology of asthma may be:
a. infection
b. a physical factor
c. an antigen-antibody reaction
d. irritants
e. all of these *Ref. 40, p. 1141*

764. Which of the following factors does not contribute to the bronchial obstruction which characterizes asthma?
a. contraction of bronchial muscle
b. swelling of the mucous membrane

c. plugging with viscid secretions
d. hyperhydration
e. increased goblet-cell secretion *Ref. 98, p. 396*

765. A disorder characterized by bilateral, intense wheezing which is unresponsive to epinephrine is?
a. croup
b. choanal atresia
c. status asthmaticus
d. bronchiolitis
e. bronchitis *Ref. 36, p. 20*

766. In which of the following diseases is wheezing the primary symptom?
a. bronchial asthma
b. croup
c. pneumonia
d. cystic fibrosis
e. kyphoscoliosis *Ref. 39, p. 314*

767. Treatment of status asthmaticus does not include:
a. oxygen
b. intravenous fluids
c. bronchodilators
d. morphine
e. aminophylline *Ref. 4, p. 85*

768. During an acute asthmatic attack:
a. airway resistance increases
b. airway resistance decreases
c. lung compliance increases
d. a and c
e. b and c *Ref. 70, p. 333*

769. A disorder characterized by recurrent paroxysmal attacks of difficult breathing is:
a. croup
b. bronchitis
c. asthma
d. bronchiolitis
e. rhinitis *Ref. 70, p. 332*

770. Which of the following factors may precipitate an asthmatic attack?
a. allergy
b. infection
c. thermal
d. psychological
e. all of these *Ref. 70, p. 329*

771. Asthma literally means:
a. difficult breathing
b. acid maker
c. wheezing
d. shortness of breath
e. obstruction *Ref. 70, p. 329*

772. Lobar pneumonia affects:
a. one lobe of the lung
b. one whole lung
c. both lungs
d. none of these
e. all of these *Ref. 98, p. 118*

773. Bilateral pneumonia is also termed:
a. lobar pneumonia
b. segmental pneumonia
c. bronchopneumonia
d. pneumonitis
e. none of these *Ref. 98, p. 112*

774. Which of the bacteria below *does not* cause pneumonia?
a. *Streptococcus pneumoniae*
b. *Staphylococcus pyogenes*
c. *Klebsiella pneumoniae*
d. *Bordetella pertussis*
e. all cause pneumonia *Ref. 98, p. 113*

775. The type of pneumothorax in which the mediastinum is shifted away from the affected side is:
a. traumatic pneumothorax
b. spontaneous pneumothorax
c. tension pneumothorax

d. open pneumothorax
e. chylothorax *Ref. 70, p. 404*

776. A pneumothorax in which the pressure is greater than atmospheric is known as:
a. traumatic pneumothorax
b. spontaneous pneumothorax
c. open pneumothorax
d. tension pneumothorax
e. chylothorax *Ref. 70, p. 404*

777. Spontaneous pneumothorax occurs most frequently in:
a. premature infants
b. children
c. premature infants and children
d. adults under 50
e. adults over 50 *Ref. 94, p. 281*

778. In children, pneumothorax usually results from:
a. a penetrating chest wound
b. foreign body
c. rupture of a bleb
d. mucous plug
e. obstruction *Ref. 25, p. 77*

779. The diagnosis of pneumothorax is made by:
a. visual examination
b. radiologic examination
c. auscultation
d. blood gas analysis
e. thoracentesis *Ref. 33, p. 124*

780. The clinical findings of pneumothorax may include:
a. cyanosis
b. tachypnea
c. grunting
d. all of these
e. b and c *Ref. 57, p. 143*

781. In cystic fibrosis:
a. RV increases
b. FRC decreases
c. TLC increases
d. RV decreases
e. none of these *Ref. 70, p. 337*

782. Cystic fibrosis involves:
a. exocrine glands
b. endocrine glands
c. an inherited genetic trait
d. a and c
e. b and c *Ref. 70, p. 334*

783. Another name for cystic fibrosis is:
a. croup
b. pectus excavatum
c. mucoviscidosis
d. bronchitis
e. bronchial asthma *Ref. 4, p. 85*

784. Cystic fibrosis presents itself clinically by:
a. coughing
b. wheezing
c. a salty taste when the child is kissed on the skin
d. all of these
e. a and b *Ref. 40, p. 1209*

785. The presence of gas in the pleural space is a disorder termed:
a. pneumomediastinum
b. pneumothorax
c. chylothorax
d. hemothorax
e. subcutaneous emphysema *Ref. 70, p. 400*

786. The procedure by which pleural fluid is obtained by aspiration is:
a. thoracentesis
b. thoracotomy
c. bronchography
d. tomography
e. bronchoscopy *Ref. 40, p. 118*

787. Pleural fluid is examined for:
a. protein content
b. specific gravity
c. presence or absence of formed cells
d. all of these
e. a and b *Ref. 40, p. 118*

788. Acute bronchitis is characterized by:
a. substernal burning discomfort
b. coughing and expectoration
c. wheezing
d. all of these
e. a and b *Ref. 70, p. 313*

789. A condition in which there is inflammation of the bronchial tree with the production of excessive mucus is:
a. bronchiolitis
b. bronchitis
c. laryngitis
d. pharyngitis
e. rhinitis *Ref. 70, p. 312*

790. Meconium-stained amniotic fluid is an indication of:
a. fetal asphyxia
b. choanal atresia
c. pneumothorax
d. Pierre Robin syndrome
e. tetralogy of Fallot *Ref. 4, p. 54*

791. A substance not found in meconium fluid is:
a. mucus
b. epithelial cells
c. bile
d. blood
e. none are present in meconium fluid

Ref. 1, p. 750

792. Meconium aspiration is often the result of:
a. prolonged labor
b. prolapsed cord
c. maternal hemorrhage
d. fetal distress
e. all of these *Ref. 33, p. 123*

793. In which of the following newborn conditions is regurgitation after feeding common?
a. bronchiolitis
b. diaphragmatic hernia
c. tracheoesophageal fistula
d. pneumothorax
e. phrenic nerve palsy *Ref. 33, p. 128*

794. A condition in which the abdominal viscera herniate into the thoracic cavity is called:
a. tracheoesophageal fistula
b. diaphragmatic hernia
c. phrenic nerve palsy
d. cardiomegaly
e. bronchopulmonary dysplasia *Ref. 33, p. 129*

795. Which of the following statements regarding transient tachypnea of the newborn is false?
a. term infants and infants born by cesarean section are at risk
b. occasionally premature infants manifest tachypnea
c. it is clinically manifested by tachypnea with dyspnea
d. the infants always require oxygen therapy
e. none of these *Ref. 33, p. 120*

796. Respiratory distress in the newborn infant may be due to:
a. cardiac anomalies
b. metabolic disorders
c. hematologic problems
d. CNS disorders
e. all of these *Ref. 33, p. 106*

797. Some common causes or manifestations of respiratory distress in the newborn infant are:

a. apnea
b. meconium aspiration
c. phrenic nerve palsy
d. all of these
e. a and b *Ref. 33, p. 106*

798. A congenital heart abnormality in which the aorta originates from the right ventricle and the pulmonary artery from the left ventricle is:

a. tetralogy of Fallot
b. transposition of the great vessels
c. anomalous venous return
d. coarctation of the aorta
e. tricuspid atresia *Ref. 40, p. 1175*

799. A congenital heart abnormality resulting in retention of the embryologic bulbar trunk is:

a. truncus arteriosus
b. ductus arteriosus
c. ligamentum nuchae
d. ventricular septal defect
e. atrial septal defect *Ref. 40, p. 1174*

800. A pediatric disorder characterized by failure of an oval hole to close between the left and right atriums of the heart is:

a. tetralogy of Fallot
b. mitral stenosis
c. patent foramen ovale
d. ductus arteriosus
e. none of these *Ref. 2, p. 6*

801. Tetralogy of Fallot is a congenital cardiovascular anomaly resulting from abnormal embryologic development of the:

a. interventricular septum
b. pulmonary artery
c. aorta
d. all of these
e. none of these *Ref. 4, p. 70*

802. An abnormal opening between the right and left ventricles is:
a. patent ductus arteriosus
b. ventricular septal defect
c. tetralogy of Fallot
d. ligamentum arteriosum
e. atrial septal defect *Ref. 40, p. 1174*

803. In the normal newborn, the ductus arteriosus degenerates to become the:
a. truncus arteriosus
b. tetralogy of Fallot
c. left atrium
d. ligamentus arteriosum
e. interventricular septum *Ref. 40, p. 1173*

804. The persistence of a fetal connection between the pulmonary artery and the aorta is termed:
a. patent ductus arteriosus
b. atrial septal defect
c. ventricular septal defect
d. coarctation of the aorta
e. tetralogy of Fallot *Ref. 40, p. 1173*

805. The etiology of congenital heart disease may be:
a. fetal infection
b. maternal infection
c. maternal dietary deficiencies
d. hereditary
e. all of these *Ref. 40, p. 1172*

806. The surgical anastomosis between the aorta and the left pulmonary artery is called a:
a. Potts-Smith-Gibson procedure
b. Brock's procedure
c. Blalock-Taussig shunt
d. Mustard's procedure
e. none of these *Ref. 40, p. 1181*

807. The surgical anastomosis between the right subclavian artery and the right pulmonary artery is a:
a. Rashkind procedure
b. Mustard's procedure

c. Blalock-Taussig shunt
d. Blalock-Hanlon procedure
e. Brock's procedure *Ref. 40, p. 1181*

808. The surgical anastomosis between the posterior lateral aspect of the ascending aorta and the right pulmonary artery is a:
a. Waterston shunt
b. Blalock-Taussig shunt
c. Potts-Smith-Gibson procedure
d. Brock's procedure
e. Mustard's procedure *Ref. 40, p. 1180*

809. Complete correction of transposition of the great vessels is performed by a:
a. Rashkind procedure
b. Blalock-Hanlon procedure
c. Mustard's procedure
d. Potts-Smith-Gibson procedure
e. Brock's procedure *Ref. 40, p. 1179*

810. A Rashkind procedure refers to:
a. creation of an atrial septal defect with a balloon catheter
b. creation of a ventricular septal defect with a balloon catheter
c. surgical correction of a ventricular septal defect
d. correction of a patent ductus arteriosus
e. none of these *Ref. 40, p. 1179*

811. The purpose of a Blalock-Hanlon procedure is:
a. surgical correction of an atrial septal defect
b. surgical creation of an atrial septal defect
c. surgical removal of the atrial septum
d. surgical addition to the atria
e. none of these *Ref. 40, p. 1179*

812. If a coarctation of the descending aorta is proximal to the ductus arteriosus it is called:
a. hypoductal
b. hyperductal
c. preductal
d. postductal
e. aductal *Ref. 40, p. 117*

813. In tricuspid atresia, the lungs may receive blood through:
a. bronchial vessels
b. a small ventricular septal defect
c. a patent ductus arteriosus
d. all of these
e. b and c *Ref. 40, p. 1175*

814. A congenital heart abnormality characterized by a small right ventricle, large left ventricle and, usually, diminished pulmonary circulation is:
a. subaortic stenosis
b. patent ductus arteriosus
c. ventricular septal defect
d. tricuspid atresia
e. transposition of great vessels *Ref. 40, p. 1175*

815. A congenital heart abnormality characterized by a narrowed aortic lumen is:
a. tricuspid atresia
b. tetralogy of Fallot
c. subaortic stenosis
d. coarctation of the aorta
e. ventricular septal defect *Ref. 40, p. 1174*

816. An abnormal opening between the right and left atria is a:
a. ventricular septal defect
b. atrial septal defect
c. truncus arteriosus
d. subaortic stenosis
e. anomalous venous return *Ref. 40, p. 1175*

817. The cardinal clinical features suggesting the presence of heart failure in the newborn are:

a. dyspnea and hepatomegaly
b. dyspnea, tachycardia and venous congestion
c. tachycardia, hepatomegaly and venous congestion
d. tachycardia and venous congestion
e. dyspnea, tachycardia, hepatomegaly and venous congestion *Ref. 31, p. 878*

818. In a child with congenital heart disease, cyanosis can be visualized by checking the:

a. lips
b. tongue
c. mucous membranes
d. nail beds
e. all of these *Ref. 40, p. 1181*

In column A are listed various diseases. In column B are found the definitions. Match column A and column B.

Column A

819. _____ cystic fibrosis *Ref. 4, p. 85*

820. _____ kyphoscoliosis *Ref. 4, p. 80*

821. _____ asthma *Ref. 4, p. 81*

822. _____ pneumonia *Ref. 70, p. 340*

823. _____ bronchiolitis *Ref. 4, p. 80*

824. _____ bronchitis *Ref. 70, p. 312*

825. _____ laryngitis *Ref. 99, p. 1188*

826. _____ croup *Ref. 4, p. 79*

827. _____ choanal atresia *Ref. 4, p. 61*

828. _____ bacterial pneumonia *Ref. 70, p. 341*

Column B

a. an inflammation of the membrane that lines the bronchial tubes

b. an inflammation of the trachea and the bronchi

c. an acute inflammation of the smallest bronchi, occurring in infants and small children

d. curvature of the spine

e. an acute infection which results in inflammation of the lung that fills the lung tissues and air spaces with liquid matter (consolidation)

f. a disease caused by *Streptococcus*, *Staphylococcus*, *Klebsiella*, and *Hemophilus influenzae*

g. a hereditary disorder

h. recurrent attacks of shortness of breath; from the Greek word for panting

i. an inflammation of the larynx

j. unilateral or bilateral nasal obstruction

SECTION 5

Oxygen Administration and Pulmonary Function Testing

For each of the questions select the *one* most appropriate answer.

829. Oxygen is:
a. colorless, odorless and tasteless
b. an element which does not burn
c. a diatomic molecule
d. all of these
e. a and c *Ref. 26, p. 251*

830. The atomic weight of oxygen is:
a. 8
b. 12
c. 16
d. 32
e. 48 *Ref. 85, p. 136*

831. The molecular weight of oxygen is:
a. 8
b. 12
c. 16
d. 32
e. 48 *Ref. 85, p. 69*

832. The critical temperature of oxygen is:
a. −118.8 C
b. −181.1 F
c. −174.6 C
d. a and b
e. a and c *Ref. 85, p. 69*

833. The density of oxygen is:
a. 1.429 gm/L
b. 1.619 gm/L
c. 1.819 gm/L
d. 1.929 gm/L
e. 2.649 gm/L *Ref. 26, p. 251*

834. Which of the following statements are false concerning oxygen?
a. oxygen is a monatomic molecule
b. oxygen was named by Priestley
c. oxygen was discovered by Lavoisier
d. oxygen supports combustion and is flammable
e. all of the statements are false *Ref. 85, p. 69*

835. The most frequent indication for oxygen administration to newborn infants is:
a. hemoglobinemia
b. RDS
c. cyanosis
d. asphyxia neonatorum
e. apnea *Ref. 25, p. 46*

836. Oxygen is not indicated in the newborn who has:
a. asphyxia neonatorum
b. RDS
c. asthma
d. shock
e. pneumothorax *Ref. 25, p. 46*

837. When oxygen is administered to an infant or small child, it should be ordered by:
a. flow rate
b. duration
c. liter flow
d. percent desired
e. FE_{O_2} *Ref. 33, p. 109*

838. The most common method of oxygen administration in the neonate is the:
a. hood
b. nasal cannula

c. simple mask
d. partial rebreather
e. face tent *Ref. 100, p. 54*

839. Which of the following is important when administering oxygen to an infant?
a. the concentration of oxygen
b. the age of the infant
c. the duration of oxygen administration
d. all of these
e. a and c *Ref. 93, p. 19*

840. Whenever oxygen is administered to an infant:
a. it should be checked hourly
b. blood gases should be performed
c. the concentration should be analyzed
d. the data should be carefully recorded
e. all of these *Ref. 3, p. 93*

841. In a newborn infant, oxygen may be toxic to the eyes and to the:
a. heart
b. lungs
c. liver
d. kidneys
e. stomach *Ref. 3, p. 94*

842. Oxygen which is administered unheated to an infant:
a. increases oxygen consumption
b. reduces tissue hypoxia
c. eliminates the possibility of infection
d. assures adequate humidification
e. increases body temperature *Ref. 4, p. 91*

843. The administration of unheated oxygen to the face of an infant does not:
a. result in increased oxygen consumption
b. cause a low relative humidity of the inspired gas
c. cause trigeminal nerve stimulation
d. result in decreased oxygen consumption
e. have any effect *Ref. 29, p. 459*

844. By what method can oxygen not be delivered to an infant?

a. endotracheal tube
b. mask
c. catheter
d. hood
e. incubator *Ref. 3, p. 93*

845. Any infant requiring oxygen therapy for respiratory distress longer than 1 hour after birth should have a:

a. W.B.C. and differential
b. chest x-ray
c. complete c.b.c.
d. mechanical ventilator available
e. increased $F_{I_{O_2}}$ *Ref. 4, p. 61*

846. If a comatose infant or child requires oxygen therapy, the appropriate method is:

a. nasal catheter
b. oxygen mask
c. oxygen croupette or tent
d. oxygen cannula
e. tracheostomy mask *Ref. 25, p. 100*

847. In general, when oxygen is administered to a child, the effect should be:

a. decreasing restlessness
b. decreasing respiratory distress
c. improvement of color
d. improvement in vital signs
e. all of these *Ref. 40, p. 1096*

848. A possible complication of oxygen administration is:

a. nausea
b. substernal distress
c. carbon dioxide narcosis
d. retrolental fibroplasia
e. all of these *Ref. 40, p. 1095*

849. To measure the effectiveness of oxygen administration, the clinician should:

a. look for relief of cyanosis

b. measure Pa_{O_2}
c. measure PA_{O_2}
d. a and b
e. a and c *Ref. 40, p. 1095*

850. When an infant or small child is being weaned from oxygen, the clinician should watch for:
a. pulse elevation
b. tachypnea
c. cyanosis
d. all of these
e. none of these *Ref. 40, p. 1097*

851. Which of the following statements is false concerning oxygen administration in newborns?
a. the duration of oxygen administration should be as short as possible
b. the oxygen concentration should be analyzed and recorded hourly
c. oxygen should be routinely administered to healthy premature infants
d. oxygen should always be warmed and humidified
e. oxygen should be ordered by percent and not by liter flow *Ref. 33, p. 108*

852. The administration of high oxygen concentrations to an infant can result in:
a. retrolental fibroplasia
b. pulmonary hemorrhage
c. bronchopulmonary dysplasia
d. all of these
e. a and c *Ref. 33, p. 108*

853. Oxygen enrichment of the inspired air may improve or correct hypoxemia when it is due to:
a. diffusion defects
b. alveolar hyperventilation
c. low ventilation-perfusion ratios
d. all of these
e. a and c *Ref. 36, p. 4*

854. In newborn infants the Pa_{O_2} should be maintained between:

a. 20–40 mm Hg
b. 40–60 mm Hg
c. 50–80 mm Hg
d. 60–100 mm Hg
e. 80–100 mm Hg *Ref. 33, p. 111*

855. The simplest, most economical and most effective method of administering 21%–100% oxygen to an infant is:

a. nasal cannula
b. CPAP apparatus
c. oxygen hood
d. incubator
e. mechanical ventilator *Ref. 33, p. 110*

856. When breathing room air at sea level, FI_{O_2} is approximately:

a. 159 mm Hg
b. 150 mm Hg
c. 104 mm Hg
d. 95–100 mm Hg
e. 40–60 mm Hg *Ref. 101, p. 1071*

857. Increasing the inspired oxygen concentration by 10% means increasing the inspired oxygen tension approximately:

a. 20 mm Hg
b. 35 mm Hg
c. 50 mm Hg
d. 65 mm Hg
e. 75 mm Hg *Ref. 28, p. 92*

858. The Olympic Oxyhood has which of the following available features?

a. controlled temperature monitoring
b. inlets for I.V.'s
c. no seal required between neck and head
d. availability for high oxygen concentration
e. all of these *Ref. 100, pp. 54–55*

859. The Olympic Oxyhood is available in what sizes?
a. large, medium, small, infant
b. medium, small
c. medium, small, infant
d. large, medium, small
e. none of these *Ref. 100, p. 55*

860. The Olympic Oxyhood will fit infants in what weight range?
a. 4–20 lb
b. 2–18 lb
c. 2–20 lb
d. 4–18 lb
e. 4–24 lb *Ref. 100, p. 55*

861. The special feature of the Olympic Oxyhood is that it:
a. is clear so you can see the infant
b. is lightweight
c. requires no seal around the infant's neck
d. can maintain high concentrations of oxygen
e. all of these *Ref. 100, p. 55*

862. A disadvantage of oxygen hoods is:
a. FI_{O_2} is difficult to control
b. humidity delivered is substandard
c. inspired gas temperature cannot be controlled
d. the hood must be removed for feeding
e. the infant's face is not visible *Ref. 4, p. 96*

863. A hood is often used in conjunction with an incubator to:
a. increase the relative humidity
b. provide a more constant temperature to the infant
c. protect the infant from variations of inspired oxygen
d. stimulate the thermal receptors in the infant's face
e. all of these *Ref. 4, p. 92*

864. The flow rate necessary to prevent CO_2 accumulation in a hood is:
a. 2 liters per minute
b. 3 liters per minute
c. 5 liters per minute
d. 6 liters per minute
e. 8 liters per minute *Ref. 25, p. 54*

865. Which of the following is not a complication of positive-pressure hoods or plastic head bags?
a. cooling of the face
b. high sound levels
c. facial pressure necrosis
d. fluctuations of oxygen concentrations
e. all of these *Ref. 102, pp. 131, 170*

866. An incubator provides:
a. controlled environment
b. reverse isolation
c. heat balance
d. humidity
e. all of these *Ref. 3, p. 62*

867. Transport incubators should be designed and equipped to provide:
a. warmth
b. visibility
c. portability
d. storage for oxygen and electrical power
e. all of these *Ref. 3, pp. 86–87*

868. When administering oxygen by croupette or Isolette, it is recommended that $F_{I_{O_2}}$ be monitored at least:
a. every hour
b. every 2 hours
c. every 4 hours
d. every 8 hours
e. every 24 hours *Ref. 3, p. 92*

869. The purpose of providing high relative humidity to an infant in an incubator is to:
a. prevent water loss from the skin

b. prevent water loss from the respiratory tract
c. prevent secretions in the respiratory tract from drying
d. all of these
e. b and c *Ref. 25, p. 105*

870. The relative humidity in incubators should be between:
a. 30%–45%
b. 50%–65%
c. 65%–75%
d. 80%–90%
e. 90%–100% *Ref. 3, p. 90*

871. In an Isolette, if the red flag is up, what does this indicate?
a. the oxygen supply is inadequate
b. the oxygen supply is unplugged
c. oxygen is in use
d. more than 40% oxygen is being used
e. it could mean *any* of these things

Ref. 100, p. 58

872. A radiant warmer is used in preference to an incubator whenever:
a. isolation is necessary
b. complete access to the infant is needed
c. precise temperature control is mandatory
d. high oxygen concentrations are required
e. an x-ray will be taken *Ref. 25, p. 109*

873. A croup tent should:
a. be capable of operation from room air or oxygen
b. be cool
c. provide adequate humidity
d. allow usage in both infants and children
e. all of these *Ref. 4, p. 97*

874. The concentration of oxygen attainable in a croup tent is:
a. 21%–25%
b. 25%–30%
c. 30%–40%
d. 30%–50%
e. over 50% *Ref. 25, p. 103*

875. Under ideal conditions, the temperature within a croup tent is:
a. the same as the room temperature
b. 3 F cooler than the room temperature
c. 7 F cooler than the room temperature
d. 12 F cooler than the room temperature
e. 16 F cooler than the room temperature
Ref. 25, p. 97

876. Oxygen croup tent canopies should:
a. be made of slow-burning material
b. have a No Smoking sign on them
c. have animals on them
d. all of these
e. a and b *Ref. 103, pp. 62–63*

877. Oxygen croup tent canopies should be constructed of:
a. cellulose acetate
b. nitrocellulose
c. pyroxylin
d. a and b
e. b and c *Ref. 103, p. 64*

878. Which of the following is not a safety feature of a croup tent?
a. the canopy
b. the plastic water reservoir
c. the grounded plug
d. the humidity control
e. the oxygen fitting *Ref. 103, pp. 27, 63–64, 71*

879. In which of the following situations should mist-tent therapy be discontinued?
a. croup
b. patients with voluminous secretions

c. bronchiolitis
d. all of these
e. none of these *Ref. 25, p. 75*

880. Which of the following is *not* a possible function of an oxygen croup tent?
a. to administer oxygen therapy
b. to control temperature
c. to administer humidity therapy
d. to administer helium-oxygen therapy
e. none of these *Ref. 25, p. 103*

881. In order to maintain an adequate oxygen concentration in a croup tent, the clinician should:
a. use a tight-fitting canopy
b. avoid opening the canopy
c. analyze the FI_{O_2}
d. use the smallest-size canopy possible
e. all of these *Ref. 25, pp. 103–104*

882. The possible shortcomings of placing a small child in a high-humidity croup tent are:
a. claustrophobia
b. anxiety
c. confinement
d. all of these
e. none of these *Ref. 25, p. 114*

883. An infant mask should:
a. conform to the patient's face easily
b. possess a soft rim
c. have 10–15 ml deadspace
d. all of these
e. a and b *Ref. 63, p. 241*

884. In children a soft vinyl mask should be used to:
a. prevent CO_2 accumulation
b. prevent pressure necrosis
c. relieve anoxia
d. reduce discomfort
e. administer helium-oxygen mixtures
Ref. 25, p. 100

885. An oxygen mask should:
a. be easily cleaned and stored
b. have adjustable head straps
c. always have a reservoir
d. be designed so that CO_2 accumulation is minimal
e. be made of indestructible material

Ref. 25, p. 100

886. A large adult mask should not be used to administer oxygen to children because:
a. children are prone to vomiting
b. the risk of aspiration is increased
c. the space inside the mask is added deadspace
d. it is uncomfortable
e. high concentrations cannot be achieved

Ref. 25, p. 100

887. A child has a massive postoperative atelectasis. Oxygen by mask is administered with a well-fitting reservoir-type mask at a flow rate of 15 liters per minute. Despite this, the patient remains cyanotic. The reason is:
a. the patient should be on a ventilator
b. the patient is probably anemic and, thus, there is not enough hemoglobin to pick up the oxygen
c. an inadequate amount of oxygen is being given to the patient
d. the atelectatic lung still has pulmonary circulation, although ventilation is completely shut off, and thus acts as a large venous shunt
e. the patient's peak inspiratory flow rate is not being met *Ref. 28, p. 69*

888. The type of face mask which is designed to administer precisely controlled low oxygen concentrations is the:
a. simple mask
b. Venturi mask
c. partial rebreathing mask
d. non-rebreathing mask
e. tracheostomy mask *Ref. 40, p. 131*

889. Standard available FI_{O_2} settings with Puritan all-purpose nebulizers are:
a. ambient–60%–100%
b. ambient–40%–100%
c. 40%–60%–100%
d. 40%–70%–100%
e. 40%–80%–100% *Ref. 71, p. 102*

890. Standard available FI_{O_2} settings with Ohio deluxe nebulizers are:
a. ambient–40%–100%
b. ambient–60%–100%
c. 40%–50%–100%
d. 40%–60%–100%
e. 40%–70%–100% *Ref. 104*

891. The Olympic tracheostomy button and the Kistner valve are similar because they both:
a. are designed to maintain the stoma
b. have one-way valves permitting inhalation only
c. are used in preference to endotracheal intubation
d. a and b
e. a and c *Ref. 105*

892. The primary purpose of the Angel Frame is:
a. traction
b. ventilator tubing support
c. to decrease mobility
d. an infant bed
e. CPAP administration *Ref. 25, p. 132*

893. A major disadvantage of the use of cones and funnels to deliver oxygen to neonates is:
a. lack of adequate humidity
b. difficulty of connecting tubing to it
c. lack of precision oxygen delivery
d. inability to accurately measure the FI_{O_2}
e. all of these *Ref. 4, p. 93*

894. Generally speaking, flow rates in excess of 6 liters per minute are not recommended when using a nasal cannula because:

a. flows this high may produce inactivation of nasopharyngeal cilia
b. flows this high have been found to be a contributing factor to pain in the frontal sinuses
c. flows this high have been found to cause excessive drying of the lower respiratory tract
d. flows this high may produce a Venturi effect and cause entrainment of room air through the nostrils
e. the concentration of oxygen attainable is not high enough *Ref. 26, p. 266*

895. Water in the gaseous state is called:

a. molecular water
b. water vapor
c. saturated water
d. all of these
e. a and b *Ref. 28, p. 11*

896. The percentage of water vapor in air compared with the amount which the air is capable of holding if fully saturated is called the:

a. water vapor pressure
b. % saturation
c. relative humidity
d. absolute humidity
e. temperature-humidity index *Ref. 26, p. 14*

897. The primary reason for humidifying inspired gases is:

a. to soothe irritated mucous membranes
b. to combat systemic dehydration
c. to thin and loosen secretions
d. to deliver droplets to the peripheral areas of the lungs
e. to eliminate drying of the tracheobronchial mucosa *Ref. 48, p. 120*

898. The administration of dry gases does not result in:

a. dehydration of the respiratory mucosa
b. depression of the ciliary motion

c. thick, dry, tenacious secretions
d. decreased resistance to ventilation
e. none of these *Ref. 106, p. 230*

899. To saturate a dry gas at 37 C, ______ mg of water must be added per liter of gas.
a. 44
b. 53
c. 60
d. 78
e. 90 *Ref. 107, p. 105*

900. The drying of secretions in an artificial airway should never occur if:
a. humidification is adequate
b. suction is effective
c. oxygen concentration is monitored
d. all of these
e. a and b *Ref. 108, p. 145*

901. The most common danger of humidity and nebulization therapy in infants is:
a. respiratory tract burns
b. infection
c. overhydration
d. all of these
e. b and c *Refs. 4, p. 104; 25, p. 114*

902. Which of the following is *not* a consequence of breathing air which is too warm and too moist?
a. a loss in the specific airway resistance
b. hyperthermia
c. water overload
d. hypoxia
e. bronchopneumonia *Ref. 109, p. 221*

903. Heated nebulizers are used principally to:
a. decrease relative humidity
b. increase the concentration of medication delivered
c. propel water vapor to the patient
d. increase the amount of liquid delivered to the airways
e. none of these *Ref. 71, p. 100*

904. The formula to convert F to C is:

a. C = 5/9 F (+ 32)
b. 5 F = 9 C + 160
c. C = 9/5 (F − 32)
d. C = 9/5 F (+ 32)
e. b and d *Ref. 26, p. 449*

905. Using the previous formula, what would be a child's temperature in Fahrenheit if the Centigrade thermometer read 39 C?

a. 98.6 F
b. 100.2 F
c. 102.5 F
d. 104 F
e. 105 F *Ref. 26, p. 449*

906. A heated nebulizer used in a neonatal ICU should be changed every:

a. 4 hours
b. 8 hours
c. 16 hours
d. 24 hours
e. 72 hours *Ref. 3, p. 50*

907. What is the humidity deficit if a patient is breathing air containing 33 mg/L?

a. 20.8 mg/L
b. 15.0 mg/L
c. 25.8 mg/L
d. 11.0 mg/L
e. 43.0 mg/L *Ref. 26, p. 206*

908. The purpose of an immersion heater in a nebulizer is to:

a. decrease relative humidity
b. eliminate a humidity deficit
c. increase relative humidity
d. eliminate dissemination of water bacteria
e. propel water vapor to the patient

Ref. 71, p. 100

909. Neonates and infants are very susceptible to effects of infection, particularly if debilitated. To help prevent infection in an infant, clinicians should:
a. wash their hands between patients
b. wash their hands before and after handling infants
c. preferably wear gowns
d. change equipment frequently
e. all of these *Ref. 3, pp. 41, 50, 107*

910. An organism which is not likely to contaminate respiratory therapy equipment is:
a. *Streptococcus fecalis*
b. *Pseudomonas*
c. *Klebsiella*
d. *Aerobacter*
e. *Escherichia coli* *Ref. 110, p. 126*

911. Nebulizers, tubing and water traps should be cleaned and sterilized every:
a. hour
b. 4 hours
c. 8 hours
d. 12 hours
e. 24 hours *Ref. 3, p. 50*

912. The type of water which should be used for refilling the water reservoir of incubators and nebulizers is:
a. tap water
b. cold water
c. autoclaved water
d. sterile, distilled water
e. c and d *Ref. 3, p. 50*

913. What size oxygen cylinder is used most often in transport vehicles?
a. "D" size
b. "E" size
c. "F" size
d. "G" size
e. "H" size *Ref. 41, p. 44*

914. What size oxygen cylinder is used most often with transport incubators?

a. "D" size
b. "E" size
c. "F" size
d. "G" size
e. "H" size *Ref. 41, p. 44*

915. To check the accuracy of an oxygen blender one should:

a. check the wall pressure hourly
b. measure the Pa_{O_2}
c. use an oxygen analyzer
d. draw arterial blood gases
e. do frequent hemoglobin and hematocrit measurements *Ref. 55, p. 313*

916. Most oxygen blenders are accurate as long as wall air and oxygen pressures are at:

a. 40 p.s.i.
b. 45 p.s.i.
c. 50 p.s.i.
d. 55 p.s.i.
e. 60 p.s.i. *Ref. 55, p. 313*

917. A patient is receiving oxygen through a blender that delivers 50% oxygen. What is the approximate partial pressure of oxygen (atmospheric pressure at sea level) delivered to the patient?

a. 100 mm Hg
b. 159 mm Hg
c. 380 mm Hg
d. 500 mm Hg
e. 760 mm Hg *Ref. 26, p. 11*

918. A side-effect which the clinician who administers CO_2/O_2 mixtures should watch for is:

a. hyperthermia
b. bronchial dilation
c. air hunger
d. palpitation
e. bradypnea *Ref. 26, p. 280*

919. The usual pressure of oxygen at the wall outlet of a piping system is:
a. 50 mm Hg
b. 50 cm H_2O
c. 50 torr
d. 50 p.s.i.
e. 50 atmospheres *Ref. 26, p. 237*

920. The Wright spirometer can be used to measure:
a. V_T
b. MV
c. vital capacity
d. all of these
e. a and b *Ref. 111, pp. 60–61*

921. The Beckman oxygen analyzer works on the principle of:
a. partial pressures
b. thermal conductivity
c. paramagnetism
d. fuel cells
e. thermistors *Ref. 71, p. 88*

922. The Beckman oxygen analyzer does *not* incorporate a:
a. sampling tube
b. drying chamber
c. fuel cell
d. aspirator bulb
e. oxygen concentration scale *Ref. 71, p. 87*

923. The normal color of silica gel in the Beckman oxygen analyzer is:
a. blue
b. pink
c. orange
d. red
e. green *Ref. 112, p. 208*

924. The purpose of silica gel in the Beckman oxygen analyzer is to:

a. absorb moisture
b. add moisture
c. remove carbon dioxide
d. allow calibration of the source gas
e. none of these *Ref. 112, p. 208*

925. When the silica gel crystals in the Beckman oxygen analyzer turn ______, they should be changed.

a. blue
b. pink
c. orange
d. red
e. green *Ref. 112, p. 208*

926. As altitude increases, the percentage of oxygen concentration shown on the Beckman oxygen analyzer will be:

a. higher than the actual concentration
b. lower than the actual concentration
c. unaffected
d. higher above 5000 ft
e. lower below 5000 ft *Ref. 112, p. 208*

927. If a clinician is giving 10 liters-per-minute flow via CPAP to a patient and 5 liters per minute is O_2 and 5 liters per minute is air, what is the concentration of oxygen?

a. 30%
b. 40%
c. 50%
d. 60%
e. 80% *Ref. 25, p. 133*

928. A common problem which can occur during transportation of newborns is:

a. apnea
b. cyanosis
c. regurgitation
d. aspiration
e. all of these *Ref. 33, p. 31*

929. IPPB is generally *not* used to:
a. increase alveolar ventilation
b. increase minute ventilation
c. elevate arterial oxygen saturation
d. increase cardiac output
e. reduce arterial carbon dioxide tension

Ref. 26, p. 405

930. For best results, the patient receiving an IPPB treatment should be:
a. prone
b. supine
c. seated upright
d. in Trendelenburg's position
e. lying sideways *Ref. 26, p. 406*

931. Indications for IPPB include:
a. bronchitis
b. asthma
c. bronchiectasis
d. pneumonia
e. all of these *Ref. 26, p. 406*

932. IPPB affects the cardiovascular system by:
a. increasing venous return
b. decreasing oxygen saturation
c. increasing cardiac output
d. decreasing venous return
e. increasing the stroke volume *Ref. 48, p. 231*

933. Orders for IPPB therapy should include all but which one of the following?
a. duration of treatment
b. frequency of treatment
c. medication to be used
d. amount of medication
e. sensitivity setting *Ref. 48, p. 225*

934. The three general indications for aerosol therapy include all but:
a. relief of bronchospasm
b. sputum induction
c. humidification of the inspired gas
d. mobilization of secretions
e. all of these *Ref. 26, p. 188–210*

935. When administering continuous ultrasonic therapy to an infant, the clinician should make sure:
a. the reservoir bottle does not run out
b. the patient does not become overhydrated
c. the patient is weighed frequently
d. that proper infection-control procedures are instituted and maintained
e. all of these *Ref. 110, p. 125*

936. Continuous ultrasonic nebulization with an unmodified device should not be used:
a. in patients with pulmonary edema
b. in newborns
c. in overhydrated patients
d. all of these
e. none of these *Ref. 91, p. 36*

937. The most common organism contaminating ultrasonic nebulizers is:
a. *Pseudomonas aeruginosa*
b. *Staphylococcus aureus*
c. *Serratia marcescens*
d. *Hemophilus influenzae*
e. *Klebsiella bacillus* *Ref. 113, p. 719*

938. The output of an ultrasonic nebulizer is determined by:
a. frequency
b. amplitude
c. resistance
d. modulation
e. none of these *Ref. 71, p. 96*

939. The particle size of a resultant aerosol from ultrasonic nebulization is determined by:
a. frequency
b. amplitude
c. resistance
d. modulation
e. all of these *Ref. 71, p. 96*

940. The frequency of most commercially available ultrasonic nebulizers is ______ megacycles:
a. 1.25
b. 1.30
c. 1.35
d. 1.40
e. 1.45 *Ref. 26, p. 223*

941. The ceramic disk which vibrates and changes one type of energy to another type of energy is a:
a. condenser
b. module
c. transducer
d. generator
e. vibrator *Ref. 26, p. 224*

942. The definition of CPPB is:
a. mechanical ventilation against a threshold resistance
b. the same as CPAP
c. a spontaneously breathing infant with positive pressure on inspiration
d. nonventilator breathing against a threshold resistance
e. b and d *Ref. 111, p. 211*

943. Another name for CPAP is:
a. IPPB
b. PEEP
c. CPPB
d. CNP
e. IPPV *Ref. 4, p. 173*

944. CPAP can be applied to an infant by means of:
a. face mask
b. nasotracheal tube
c. nasal prongs
d. sealed head chamber
e. all of these *Ref. 114, p. 85*

945. CPAP may not be applied via:
a. mask
b. endotracheal tube
c. nasal prongs
d. face tent
e. plastic head chamber *Ref. 114, p. 85*

946. CPAP most accurately describes
a. continuous pressure on inspiration
b. continuous pressure on exhalation
c. 0–10 cm PEEP
d. continuous pressure throughout the respiratory cycle
e. none of these *Ref. 4, p. 173*

947. The use of CPAP:
a. decreases FRC
b. prevents microatelectasis
c. increases A-a gradient
d. is routine in a spontaneously breathing infant
e. is only applicable for a spontaneously breathing infant *Ref. 25, p. 61*

948. The criteria for instituting continuous positive airway pressure is:
a. hypoxia
b. apnea
c. hypoxia and apnea
d. cyanosis
e. hypoxia and cyanosis *Ref. 35, p. 247*

949. CPAP is usually used in a range of:
a. 0–5 cm H_2O
b. 0–15 cm H_2O
c. 5–15 cm H_2O

d. 5–20 cm H_2O
e. 0–25 cm H_2O *Ref. 25, p. 63*

950. Every CPAP system should possess a:
a. pressure recorder
b. safety pop-off
c. reservoir bag
d. humidified air-oxygen system
e. all of these *Ref. 115, p. 1334*

951. In a CPAP system, rebreathing is prevented by:
a. the reservoir bag
b. controlling the $F_{I_{O_2}}$
c. placement of a one-way valve
d. increasing the flow rate
e. none of these *Ref. 116, p. 38*

952. The application of 3–10 cm H_2O by CPAP to a spontaneously breathing infant:
a. decreases FRC
b. decreases VC
c. increases FRC
d. increases VC
e. increases TLC *Ref. 20, p. 159*

953. Bagging an infant on CPAP is useful to:
a. manually sigh the patient
b. increase Pa_{CO_2} levels to acceptable ranges
c. reduce elevated Pa_{CO_2} levels
d. reduce the airway pressure
e. a and c *Ref. 114, p. 89*

954. According to Gregory, CPAP therapy is best used when:
a. pulmonary atelectasis ensues along with hypoxemia
b. arterial carbon dioxide tensions are low and hypoxemia is present
c. hypoxemia alone occurs
d. respiratory acidosis ensues
e. all of these *Ref. 115, p. 1334*

955. Elevated Pa_{CO_2} levels in infants receiving CPAP therapy may be treated by:
a. decreasing FI_{O_2}
b. bagging the infant
c. reducing the flow rate
d. lowering the CPAP level
e. none of these *Ref. 117, p. 410*

956. Delivery of CPAP by mask allows for:
a. ease of nursing care
b. possible skin maceration
c. prevention of intubation complications
d. all of these
e. a and c *Ref. 118, pp. 2, 4*

957. When administering CPAP by face mask:
a. the flow rate must be very low
b. a gastric decompression tube should be in place
c. the infant cannot be fed
d. b and c
e. none of these *Ref. 118, p. 1117*

958. Nasal CPAP cannot be used effectively in patients with:
a. cleft lip
b. cleft palate
c. laryngotracheal abnormalities
d. all of these
e. a and b *Ref. 21, p. 223*

959. The safety feature in the classical Gregory CPAP system is the:
a. apnea alarm
b. low pressure alarm
c. high pressure pop-off
d. oxygen alarm
e. power failure alarm *Ref. 114, p. 86*

960. The Carden valve is most directly related to:
a. anesthesia
b. resuscitation devices
c. CPPB administration

d. mechanical ventilators
e. aspiration of secretions *Ref. 119, p. 110*

961. When the Carden valve is being used, a short reservoir tube of 15 ml capacity is necessary to:
a. wash out carbon dioxide
b. reduce deadspace
c. increase the $F_{I_{O_2}}$
d. prevent entrainment of room air
e. increase the end-expiratory pressure
Ref. 119, p. 112

962. Which of the following statements concerning the Carden valve is false?
a. it is lightweight
b. it works by the Venturi principle
c. the resistance to gas flow is increased
d. the amount of deadspace is less than 2 ml
e. when gas flow is increased, end-expiratory pressure is increased *Ref. 119, p 112*

963. Which of the following infant CPAP systems incorporates an oxygen blender in its design?
a. Fluorocarbon
b. Searle
c. Bourns
d. a and b
e. b and c *Refs. 120–122*

964. In which of the following infant CPAP systems is endotracheal intubation not necessary?
a. Fluorocarbon
b. Searle
c. Bourns
d. a and b
e. b and c *Refs. 120–122*

965. The Bourns Infant CPAP system has a preset pressure pop-off at:
a. 15 cm H_2O
b. 20 cm H_2O
c. 25 cm H_2O
d. 30 cm H_2O
e. 40 cm H_2O *Ref. 122*

966. The Fluorocarbon Infant Chamber is designed for:
a. oxygen only
b. CPAP
c. CNP
d. mechanical ventilation
e. none of these *Ref. 120*

Match the symbol in column A with the appropriate definition in column B.

Column A

967. ______ VT
968. ______ FRC
969. ______ RV
970. ______ TLC
971. ______ VC
972. ______ ERV
973. ______ IC

Column B

a. amount of gas contained in the lung at the end of a maximal inspiration
b. the maximal volume of gas that can be expelled from the lungs following a maximal inspiration
c. maximum volume of gas that can be inspired from the resting expiratory level
d. volume of gas inspired or expired during each respiratory cycle
e. volume of gas remaining in the lungs at the resting expiratory level
f. volume of gas remaining in the lungs at the end of a maximal expiration
g. the maximal volume of gas that can be expired from the end-expiratory level *Ref. 25, p. 158*

974. The amount of air inhaled or exhaled during each respiratory cycle is the:
a. ERV
b. RV
c. V_T
d. IRV
e. TLC *Ref. 25, p. 138*

975. The maximum volume of gas that can be inhaled at the end of a spontaneous inspiration is the:
a. ERV
b. V_T
c. IRV
d. RV
e. FRC *Ref. 12, p. 39*

976. The maximum volume of gas that can be expired at the end of a spontaneous expiration is the:
a. ERV
b. V_T
c. IRV
d. RV
e. FRC *Ref. 12. p. 39*

977. Vital capacity is defined as the:
a. volume exhaled after a quiet inspiration
b. volume exhaled after a quiet expiration
c. largest volume of air which can be exhaled after the deepest possible inspiration
d. total volume of air in the lungs
e. TLC – FRC + IRV *Ref. 25, p. 158*

978. Residual volume refers to the gas that is left in the lungs:
a. after the deepest exhalation
b. after a quiet inspiration
c. after the deepest inspiration
d. after a quiet exhalation
e. following birth *Ref. 25, p. 158*

979. The amount of gas remaining in the lung following a maximal exhalation is:

a. V_T
b. IC
c. ERV
d. FRC
e. RV *Ref. 25, p. 158*

980. The volume in the lung at the end of a normal exhalation is called the:

a. expiratory reserve volume
b. residual volume
c. functional residual capacity
d. vital capacity
e. none of these *Ref. 39, p. 304*

981. Total lung capacity is not decreased in:

a. pulmonary edema
b. bronchiolar obstruction
c. atelectasis
d. neoplasms
e. pneumothorax *Ref. 77, p. 11*

982. The inspiratory capacity normally comprises what percent of the vital capacity?

a. 25%
b. 35%
c. 50%
d. 75%
e. 85% *Ref. 77, p. 3*

983. The expiratory reserve volume normally comprises what percent of the vital capacity?

a. 25%
b. 35%
c. 50%
d. 75%
e. 85% *Ref. 77, p. 4*

984. A decrease in vital capacity can be caused by all of the following except:
a. bronchiolar obstruction
b. pulmonary edema
c. pneumonia
d. atelectasis
e. none of these *Ref. 77, p. 2*

985. Which of the following volumes or capacities are not generally of diagnostic value?
a. IC and FRC
b. VC and RV
c. ERV and IC
d. IC, FRC and RV
e. VC and FRC *Ref. 77, p. 4*

986. Which of these values are measured indirectly?
a. V_T
b. VC
c. IC
d. RV
e. IRV *Ref. 77, p. 4*

987. Restrictive lung disease is best reflected by measuring:
a. V_T
b. VC
c. FRC
d. RV/TLC
e. TLC and RV *Ref. 25, p. 178*

988. Obstructive lung disease is best reflected by measuring:
a. VC
b. MVV
c. MMEF
d. ($FEV_{1.0}$)
e. all of these except a *Ref. 12, pp. 179–81*

989. Vital capacity is affected by:
a. anatomical structure
b. position
c. strength of the respiratory muscles
d. compliance
e. all of these *Ref. 11, p. 461*

990. Which of the following volumes provides air in the alveoli to aerate the blood even between breaths?
a. IRV
b. V_T
c. ERV
d. RV
e. none of these *Ref. 11, p. 461*

991. Closing volume plus residual volume equals:
a. expiratory reserve volume
b. closing capacity
c. functional residual volume
d. vital capacity
e. total lung capacity *Ref. 123, p. 294*

992. The critical lung volume at which airway closure is first detected is the:
a. inspiratory reserve volume
b. expiratory reserve volume
c. closing volume
d. residual volume
e. none of these *Ref. 123, p. 294*

993. Which of the following is generally given as a percent of the expired vital capacity?
a. expiratory reserve volume
b. residual volume
c. closing volume
d. tidal volume
e. inspiratory reserve volume *Ref. 123, p. 294*

994. The portion of the tidal volume which does not exchange with pulmonary blood is the:
a. anatomic deadspace
b. alveolar deadspace

c. physiologic deadspace
d. mechanical deadspace
e. none of these *Ref. 28, p. 27*

995. The volume of the conducting airways is called the:
a. anatomical deadspace
b. alveolar deadspace
c. physiologic deadspace
d. V_D/V_T ratio
e. shunt *Ref. 25, p. 151*

996. A vital capacity of less than 80% of the predicted normal is indicative of:
a. obstruction in the lung
b. restrictive disease
c. apneusis
d. males between 25 and 40 years of age
e. both obstruction and restriction
Ref. 25, p. 178

997. Residual volume is calculated by subtracting the expiratory reserve volume from the:
a. IC
b. TLC
c. FRC
d. V_T
e. VC *Ref. 25, p. 163*

998. The degree to which the epigastrium rises during inhalation is a function of the descent of the diaphragm and a rough indication of:
a. tidal volume
b. minute volume
c. respiratory rate
d. sigh volume
e. none of these *Ref. 26, p. 396*

999. Total lung capacity does not equal:

a. IC + FRC
b. VC + RV
c. IRV + V_T + ERV + RV
d. VC + ERV
e. IC + ERV + RV *Ref. 25, p. 158*

1000. Pulmonary function tests provide:

a. etiology
b. diagnosis
c. knowledge of obstruction or restriction
d. all of these
e. b and c *Ref. 25, p. 160*

1001. FRC can be determined by:

a. helium dilution
b. nitrogen washout
c. body plethysmograph
d. all of these
e. a and b *Ref. 25, p. 163*

SECTION 6

Intensive Neonatal and Pediatric Respiratory Care

For each of the questions select the *one* most appropriate answer.

1002. Ventilation is:

a. air going into and out of the lungs
b. air going from the alveoli to the capillary
c. gas exchange at the tissue level
d. equal to blood flow in the lungs
e. all of these *Ref. 26, p. 55*

1003. Hypoventilation is:

a. gas exchange in excess of 500 ml tidal volume
b. gas exchange less than 500 ml tidal volume
c. gas exchange which does not meet the metabolic demands of the body
d. breathing slowly
e. breathing deeply *Ref. 26, p. 58*

1004. Tidal volume is defined as the:

a. volume of gas inhaled per breath
b. volume of gas exhaled per breath
c. volume of gas inhaled and exhaled during each respiratory cycle
d. volume of gas remaining in the lungs after a normal breath
e. the maximum volume of gas that can be inhaled

Ref. 25, p. 158

1005. Minute volume is:
a. tidal volume + respiratory rate
b. VT × RR
c. tidal volume − anatomic deadspace × respiratory rate
d. tidal volume × respiratory rate
e. b and d *Ref. 26, p. 55*

1006. Minute volume can be calculated by knowing:
a. tidal volume and anatomical deadspace
b. respiratory rate and alveolar ventilation
c. anatomical deadspace and alveolar ventilation
d. tidal volume and respiratory rate
e. tidal volume, respiratory rate and Pa_{CO_2}
Ref. 38, p. 30

1007. The rule of thumb for determining tidal volume in the infant or child is:
a. 7 ml/kg
b. 2 ml/lb
c. 3 ml/lb
d. 7 ml/lb
e. a and c *Ref. 124, p. 96*

1008. Which of the following is the correct VT for a newborn *term* infant?
a. 50 ml
b. 100 ml
c. 15–24 ml
d. 35–45 ml
e. none of these *Ref. 25, p. 124*

1009. If the respiratory rate of a child increases and the tidal volume stays the same, the effect will be:
a. minute volume increase
b. minute volume decrease
c. minute volume unaffected
d. Pa_{CO_2} increase
e. pH decrease *Ref. 26, p. 55*

1010. Increasing the minute volume of a child on a ventilator will:

a. increase the PO_2 and decrease the pH
b. increase the PCO_2 and the pH
c. increase the pH only
d. increase the pH and decrease the PCO_2
e. none of these *Ref. 26, p. 121*

1011. The primary purpose of a mechanical ventilator is to:

a. reduce the work of breathing
b. eliminate hypoxemia
c. provide alveolar minute ventilation
d. treat and prevent hypoxia
e. reduce the FRC *Ref. 125, p. 225*

1012. Mechanical ventilators cannot be cycled by:

a. volume
b. rate
c. pressure
d. flow
e. time *Ref. 126, p. 262*

1013. A mechanical ventilator is volume-cycled when:

a. a limited amount of volume can be obtained with each preset pressure
b. the volume is preset and system pressures are variable
c. the pressure is preset and system volumes are variable
d. expiration ends with a preset volume
e. inspiration ends because of flow

Ref. 127, p. 122

1014. A mechanical ventilator is time-cycled when:

a. inspiration is ended by a preset time
b. expiration is ended by a preset time
c. the volume is preset and system pressures are variable
d. the pressure is preset and system volumes vary with time
e. the flow is preset and time varies

Ref. 124, p. 94

1015. A constant-flow generator develops which flow curve?
a. sine wave
b. square wave
c. straight line rise
d. immediate rise with a slow fall
e. slow rise with immediate fall *Ref. 48, p. 104*

1016. When a mechanical ventilator inflates a patient's lung independently of the patient's inspiratory effort, it is classified as:
a. an assistor
b. a controller
c. an assistor-controller
d. a constant-flow generator
e. a constant-pressure generator *Ref. 124, p. 93*

1017. The control on a mechanical ventilator which determines how much effort the patient must generate to initiate ventilation is:
a. flow rate
b. sensitivity
c. assist
d. sigh
e. respiratory rate *Ref. 26, p. 302*

1018. The manner in which a mechanical ventilator allows exhalation to occur may be classified as:
a. positive
b. negative
c. passive
d. retarded
e. all of these *Ref. 124, p. 94*

1019. The oxygen concentration range which should be available on a mechanical ventilator is:
a. 21%–80%
b. 30%–100%
c. 21%–100%
d. 40%–100%
e. 30%–90% *Ref. 53, p. 120*

1020. When you adjust the oxygen concentration control on a mechanical ventilator, you are regulating:

a. FI_{O_2}
b. Fa_{O_2}
c. Pi_{O_2}
d. Pa_{O_2}
e. Pe_{O_2} *Ref. 53, p. 120*

1021. The purpose of a sigh on a mechanical ventilator is to:

a. provide a periodic breath
b. cause a manual inspiration
c. increase oxygenation periodically
d. eliminate diffuse microatelectasis
e. reduce the possibility of CO_2 accumulation in the lung *Ref. 71, p. 167*

1022. A possible complication of a sigh breath is:

a. fibrosis
b. pneumothorax
c. oxygen toxicity
d. shunting
e. consolidation *Ref. 36, p. 18*

1023. Intermittent hyperinflation of patients on long-term, controlled ventilation is advisable to:

a. eliminate CO_2
b. help prevent atelectasis
c. increase venous return
d. decrease FRC
e. increase minute volume *Ref. 71, p. 167*

1024. Pressure limit controls on volume ventilators are usually designed for:

a. predetermining volume
b. predetermining flow rate
c. predetermining inspiratory time
d. predetermining expiratory time
e. predetermining maximum pressure

Ref. 128, p. 171

1025. When a pressure limit is reached, on which of the following ventilators is there an inflation hold at the airways for the remainder of the inspiratory phase?
a. Baby-Bird
b. Bourns LS 104-150 and BP 200
c. Amsterdam
d. a and b
e. b and c *Refs. 129–131*

1026. A ventilator manometer measures:
a. inspired volume
b. flow
c. resistance
d. pressure
e. expired volume *Ref. 25, p. 62*

1027. The I/E ratio refers to:
a. the length of inspiratory time
b. the relationship between flow and inspiratory time
c. the relationship between inspiratory time and expiratory time
d. the inspiratory-effort ratio
e. the length of time in total exhalation
Ref. 26, p. 379

1028. The alarm on a mechanical ventilator capable of detecting accidental disconnection is the:
a. high pressure alarm
b. low pressure alarm
c. apnea alarm
d. power failure alarm
e. oxygen alarm *Ref. 36, p. 19*

1029. If a loss of electrical power occurs during operation of an electrically powered mechanical ventilator, the alarm which will indicate the problem first is the:
a. high pressure alarm
b. apnea alarm
c. power failure alarm
d. loss-of-PEEP alarm
e. oxygen alarm *Ref. 103, p. 85*

1030. The probable cause for the high pressure alarm to sound on a mechanical ventilator is:
a. a leak in the system
b. decreased airway resistance
c. patient disconnect
d. power failure
e. increased airway resistance *Ref. 26, p. 302*

1031. Another name for a patient-disconnect alarm is:
a. low pressure alarm
b. high pressure alarm
c. power failure alarm
d. apnea alarm
e. oxygen alarm *Ref. 132, p. 14*

1032. A possible cause of the high pressure alarm on a mechanical ventilator being activated is *not*:
a. high pressure alarm set at a pressure insufficient to deliver a sigh volume
b. mucous plug in the endotracheal tube
c. endotracheal tube impinged against the carina
d. separation of the ventilator from the endotracheal tube
e. endotracheal tube slipped past carina into right main stem bronchus *Ref. 26, p. 302*

1033. The term positive pressure means pressure:
a. higher than atmospheric
b. high enough to push air into the lung
c. produced by a machine
d. inside of the chest
e. that can be measured *Ref. 111, p. 210*

1034. In which of the following methods of treatment should the pressure gauge not return to zero?
a. inspiratory plateau
b. expiratory resistance
c. retard
d. PEEP
e. none of these *Ref. 111, pp. 210–11*

1035. Positive end-expiratory pressure (PEEP) is an effective means of increasing:

a. VC
b. FRC
c. TLC
d. IRV
e. V_T *Ref. 4, p. 170*

1036. When applying positive pressure on exhalation, a possible complication is:

a. tachypnea
b. a decrease in venous return
c. hypoxemia
d. convulsions
e. hyperpnea *Ref. 111, p. 211*

1037. The inspiratory plateau-type of pressure pattern is:

a. PEEP
b. inflation hold
c. retard
d. expiratory resistance
e. none of these *Ref. 127, p. 132*

1038. An inspiratory plateau is a useful feature on a mechanical ventilator because it:

a. improves intrapulmonary mixing of gases
b. increases functional residual capacity
c. decreases the alveolar-arterial oxygen tension gradient
d. all of these
e. b and c *Ref. 35, p. 244*

1039. Which of these treatments does not occur in the expiratory phase?

a. retard
b. expiratory resistance
c. inflation hold
d. PEEP
e. none of these *Ref. 127, p. 133*

1040. In the presence of increases in flow resistance, such as with bronchospasm, a volume-cycled ventilator will:
a. alter tidal volume
b. alter delivered pressure
c. alter respiratory rate
d. all of these
e. none of these *Ref. 127, p. 122*

1041. In order to shorten the inspiratory phase of a mechanical ventilator, the clinician could:
a. use a low inspiratory flow rate
b. increase the pressure limit
c. decrease the tidal volume
d. increase the inspiratory flow rate
e. add PEEP *Ref. 127, p. 135*

In column A are listed abbreviations used to describe various forms of breathing. In column B are the definitions. Match columns A and B.

Column A	Column B
1042. ______ IPPB *Ref. 111, p. 211*	a. inspiratory plateau
1043. ______ CNP *Ref. 25, p. 63*	b. is synonymous with CPAP
1044. ______ CPAP *Ref. 111, p. 211*	c. mechanical ventilation against a threshold resistance
1045. ______ CPPB *Ref. 111, p. 211*	d. intermittent positive-pressure breathing
1046. ______ PEEP *Ref. 111, p. 211*	e. continuous negative-pressure breathing
1047. ______ inflation hold *Ref. 111, p. 211*	f. retard to exhalation
1048. ______ expiratory resistance *Ref. 111, p. 211*	g. nonventilator breathing against a threshold resistance

1049. When calculating functional VD on a mechanical ventilator you should:
a. keep the same compliance factor whenever setting up that particular ventilator
b. recalculate the factor every time you initially set up the ventilator
c. recalculate the factor when changing the tubing
d. recalculate the factor only when using other than factory-distributed tubing
e. none of these *Ref. 130*

1050. When calculating predicted VT for a neonate, you could use:
a. 2 ml/lb of body weight
b. one-half the patient's surface area divided by the body weight
c. 7 ml/kg
d. body weight divided by respiratory rate times 3 ml
e. none of these *Ref. 124, p. 96*

1051. Which of the following infant ventilators delivers a sine wave flow pattern?
a. Ohio Neonatal
b. Baby-Bird
c. Bourns LS 104-150
d. Amsterdam
e. none of these *Refs. 129–131, 133*

1052. Which of the following lung ventilators is not designed primarily for infants?
a. Amsterdam
b. Bourns LS 104-150
c. Baby-Bird
d. Ohio Neonatal
e. Monaghan 225 *Refs. 129–131, 133, 134*

1053. The Amsterdam Pediatric Ventilator is:
a. pressure-cycled
b. time-cycled
c. volume-cycled
d. pneumatically powered
e. b and c *Ref. 131, p. 128*

1054. The Baby-Bird Ventilator is:

a. volume-cycled
b. pressure-cycled
c. electrically powered
d. time-cycled
e. none of these *Ref. 129, p. 128*

1055. The Bourns LS 104-150 Infant Ventilator is classified as:

a. strictly assistor
b. strictly controller
c. assistor, controller, assistor-controller
d. assistor, controller
e. none of these *Ref. 130, p. 168*

1056. A ventilator which has a flow pattern that builds from zero to a peak at the midpoint of the inspiratory phase, then decreases steadily to zero at the end of inspiration is the:

a. Bourns LS 104-150 Infant Ventilator
b. Amsterdam Ventilator
c. Bennett MA-1 Ventilator
d. Engström ER-300 Ventilator
e. Ohio Neonatal Ventilator *Ref. 25, p. 127*

1057. An example of a ventilator which is capable of producing a square wave or sine wave flow pattern is the:

a. Ohio 550 Ventilator
b. Ohio Neonatal Ventilator
c. Servo 900 Ventilator
d. Bourns LS 104-150 Infant Ventilator
e. Baby-Bird Ventilator

Refs. 129–130, 133, 135–136

1058. Which of the following does not accurately describe the Bourns LS 104-150 Infant Ventilator?

a. assistor, controller, assistor-controller
b. pneumatically operated
c. volume-cycled
d. pressure-limited
e. constant flow generator *Ref. 130*

1059. The response time of the Bourns LS 104-150 Infant Ventilator is:

a. 82 milliseconds
b. 60 milliseconds
c. 35 milliseconds
d. 40 milliseconds
e. 50 milliseconds *Ref. 130*

1060. The range of volume delivery on the Bourns LS 104-150 Infant Ventilator is:

a. 10–100 ml
b. 10–150 ml
c. 5–100 ml
d. 5–150 ml
e. 0–150 ml *Ref. 25, p. 125*

1061. Which of the following does not apply to the Bourns LS 104-150 Infant Ventilator?

a. assistor, controller or assistor-controller
b. volume-cycled
c. pressure-limited
d. positive, passive or negative exhalation
e. electrically operated *Ref. 130*

1062. Which of the following does not apply to the Baby-Bird Ventilator?

a. time-cycled
b. pressure-limited
c. assistor-controller
d. positive or passive exhalation
e. continuous flow *Ref. 25, p. 128*

1063. The manometer on the Baby-Bird Ventilator most accurately describes the:

a. pressure at the patient's airway
b. pressure in the lung
c. pressure in the ventilator
d. pressure difference between the lung and ventilator
e. none of these *Ref. 25, pp. 128–129*

1064. Which of the following ventilators incorporates a manufacturer's slide rule for computations?
a. Bourns
b. Baby-Bird
c. Amsterdam
d. a and b
e. a and c *Refs. 129–131*

1065. Which of these mechanical ventilators incorporates an external bag in its design for manual bagging of a patient?
a. Bourns LS 104-150 Infant Ventilator
b. Amsterdam Ventilator
c. Baby-Bird Ventilator
d. Servo 900
e. a and c *Refs. 129–131, 136*

1066. In which of the following ventilators is the amount of mechanical deadspace irrelevant?
a. Bourns LS 104-150
b. Baby-Bird
c. Amsterdam
d. Ohio Neonatal
e. Bennett MA-1 *Refs. 129–131, 133, 137*

1067. An example of a ventilator which does not produce a square wave flow pattern is the:
a. Baby-Bird
b. Bourns LS 104-150
c. Ohio Neonatal
d. Emerson
e. Amsterdam *Ref. 53, p. 126*

1068. The maximum PEEP available with the Bourns BP 200 and Baby-Bird ventilators is:
a. 5 cm H_2O
b. 10 cm H_2O
c. 15 cm H_2O
d. 20 cm H_2O
e. 25 cm H_2O *Refs. 129–130*

1069. Maximum output per minute on the ultrasonic nebulizer provided with the Bourns LS 104-150 Infant Ventilator is:

a. 1 ml/min
b. 3 ml/min
c. 0.5 ml/min
d. 15 ml/min
e. 30 ml/min *Ref. 130*

1070. The Amsterdam, Bourns BP 200 and Baby-Bird ventilators are alike in which ways?

a. all are time-cycled
b. all are pneumatic
c. all have built-in oxygen blenders
d. all have controls for PEEP
e. all are sine wave flow generators

Ref. 25, p. 128

1071. Which of these infant mechanical ventilators has an external oxygen blender?

a. Bourns LS 104-150 and BP 200
b. Ohio Neonatal
c. Baby-Bird
d. a and b
e. a and c *Refs. 129–130, 133*

1072. A mechanical ventilator which does not possess a control for sighing the patient is:

a. Bourns LS 104-150
b. Baby-Bird
c. Monaghan 225
d. a and b
e. b and c *Refs. 129–130, 134*

1073. Which ventilator provides a control for expiratory resistance?

a. Bennett MA-1
b. Ohio 550
c. Monaghan 550
d. Engström ER-300
e. a and d *Ref. 25, pp. 127–128*

1074. An example of a mechanical ventilator with a fixed 1:2 I/E ratio is the:
a. Bennett MA-1
b. Engström
c. Emerson
d. Monaghan 225
e. Ohio 550 *Ref. 26, p. 298*

1075. An example of a mechanical ventilator which is time-cycled is the:
a. Baby-Bird
b. Amsterdam
c. Bourns BP 200
d. Engström
e. all of these *Ref. 25, pp. 125–129*

1076. A mechanical ventilator which does not possess the capability to assist a patient is the:
a. Bourns LS 104-150
b. Bennett MA-1
c. Monaghan 225
d. Baby-Bird
e. Gill 1 *Refs. 129–130, 134, 137–138*

1077. A mechanical ventilator which uses fluidic technology is the:
a. Monaghan 225
b. Engström ER-300
c. Emerson
d. Ohio 550
e. a and d *Ref. 132, p. 14*

1078. Which of the following does not apply to the Bennett MA-1 Ventilator?
a. volume-cycled
b. assistor, controller or assistor-controller
c. positive, passive or negative exhalation
d. constant flow generator
e. pneumatically powered *Ref. 53, p. 128*

1079. In the Bennett MA-1 Ventilator, inspiratory time is influenced by:

a. airway resistance and lung compliance
b. the preset tidal volume
c. the peak flow control
d. all of these
e. a and c *Ref. 26, p. 302*

1080. The control on a Bennett MA-1 Ventilator which determines whether the machine will be an assistor, controller, or assistor-controller is the:

a. flow rate
b. sensitivity
c. normal pressure limit
d. expiratory resistance
e. tidal volume *Ref. 26, p. 302*

1081. When the ratio alarm is activated on the Bennett MA-1, it means:

a. the pressure limit is set too low
b. the V_T is too high
c. the flow rate should be decreased
d. inspiration exceeds expiration
e. the PEEP level is not high enough

Ref. 26, p. 302

1082. When the ratio alarm is activated on the Bennett MA-1, the clinician should:

a. increase tidal volume
b. increase flow rate
c. decrease the sigh volume
d. increase the sensitivity
e. decrease the flow rate *Ref. 26, p. 302*

1083. Which control on the Bennett MA-1 governs the I/E ratio?

a. sensitivity
b. tidal volume
c. flow rate
d. respiratory rate
e. sigh volume *Ref. 26, p. 302*

1084. The number of kg in a lb is:
a. 0.45
b. 0.96
c. 1.1
d. 2.2
e. 3.3 *Ref. 26, p. 449*

1085. One cubic centimeter is equal to:
a. 0.01 ml
b. 0.010 ml
c. .10 ml
d. 1.0 ml
e. 10 ml *Ref. 90, p. 54*

1086. An example of a mechanical ventilator in which the bellows measure exhaled gas is the:
a. Ohio 560
b. Monaghan 225
c. Gill 1
d. Bennett MA-1
e. none of these *Ref. 26, p. 301*

Match the method of triggering a mechanical ventilator with the appropriate machine. There may be more than one answer.

1087. ______ Bourns LS 104-150 *Ref. 130*
1088. ______ Baby-Bird *Ref. 129*
1089. ______ Amsterdam *Ref. 131*
1090. ______ Bennett MA-1 *Ref. 137*
1091. ______ Emerson *Ref. 139*
1092. ______ Engström ER-300 *Ref. 140*
1093. ______ Monaghan 225 *Ref. 134*
1094. ______ Ohio Neonatal *Ref. 133*
1095. ______ Ohio 550 *Ref. 135*
1096. ______ Servo 900 *Ref. 136*
1097. ______ Gill 1 *Ref. 138*

a. assistor
b. controller
c. assistor-controller

Match the method of powering a mechanical ventilator with the appropriate machine.

1098. ______ Bourns LS 104-150 *Ref. 130*
1099. ______ Baby-Bird *Ref. 129*
1100. ______ Amsterdam *Ref. 131*
1101. ______ Bennett MA-1 *Ref. 137*
1102. ______ Emerson *Ref. 139*
1103. ______ Engström ER-300 *Ref. 140*
1104. ______ Monaghan 225 *Ref. 134*
1105. ______ Ohio Neonatal *Ref. 133*
1106. ______ Ohio 550 *Ref. 135*
1107. ______ Gill 1 *Ref. 138*
1108. ______ Servo 900 *Ref. 136*

a. pneumatic
b. electric

Match the peak inspiratory flows with the appropriate mechanical ventilators.

1109. ______ Bourns LS 104-150 *Ref. 130*
1110. ______ Baby-Bird *Ref. 129*
1111. ______ Amsterdam *Ref. 131*
1112. ______ Bennett MA-1 *Ref. 137*
1113. ______ Monaghan 225 *Ref. 134*
1114. ______ Ohio Neonatal *Ref. 133*
1115. ______ Ohio 550 *Ref. 135*
1116. ______ Gill 1 *Ref. 138*
1117. ______ Servo 900 *Ref. 136*
1118. ______ Engström ER-300 *Ref. 140*

a. 120 liters per minute
b. continuous flow
c. accelerating flow

d. 100 liters
per minute
e. 12 liters per
minute

Match the appropriate flow patterns with these various mechanical ventilators. There may be more than one answer.

1119. ______ Bourns LS 104-150 *Ref. 130*
1120. ______ Baby-Bird *Ref. 129*
1121. ______ Amsterdam *Ref. 131*
1122. ______ Bennett MA-1 *Ref. 137*
1123. ______ Emerson *Ref. 139*
1124. ______ Engström ER-300 *Ref. 140*
1125. ______ Monaghan 225 *Ref. 134*
1126. ______ Ohio Neonatal *Ref. 133*
1127. ______ Ohio 550 *Ref. 135*
1128. ______ Gill 1 *Ref. 138*
1129. ______ Servo 900 *Ref. 136*

a. square wave
b. sine wave

Match the maximum sigh volumes with the appropriate mechanical ventilator.

1130. ______ Bourns LS 104-150 *Ref. 130*
1131. ______ Baby-Bird *Ref. 129*
1132. ______ Amsterdam *Ref. 131*
1133. ______ Bennett MA-1 *Ref. 137*
1134. ______ Emerson *Ref. 139*
1135. ______ Engström ER-300 *Ref. 140*
1136. ______ Monaghan 225 *Ref. 134*
1137. ______ Ohio Neonatal *Ref. 133*
1138. ______ Ohio 550 *Ref. 135*
1139. ______ Gill 1 *Ref. 138*
1140. ______ Servo 900 *Ref. 136*

a. none
b. two consecutive tidal volumes
c. 2100 ml
d. 2000 ml
e. 2200 ml

1141. The purpose of CNP therapy is to:
a. increase TLC
b. reduce ERV
c. increase FRC
d. decrease V_T
e. decrease VC *Ref. 132, p. 162*

1142. In which situations should CNP be avoided:
a. in air trapping
b. meconium aspiration
c. pneumothorax
d. all of these
e. none of these *Ref. 132, p. 164*

1143. Which of the following is not a disadvantage of using CNP in infants?
a. restricted access to the infant
b. loss of negative pressure when infants require care

c. frequent endotracheal tube problems
d. difficulty in moving patients in and out of the unit
e. all are disadvantages *Ref. 141, pp. 128, 167*

1144. The two potential dangers of negative expiratory pressure are:
a. pulmonary edema
b. air trapping
c. decreased venous return
d. a and b
e. a and c *Ref. 26, pp. 345–46*

1145. Intermittent mandatory ventilation (IMV) is:
a. IPPB with PEEP
b. a technique used with CPAP
c. continuous flow breathing
d. continuous flow breathing with periodic machine breaths
e. continuous flow breathing with periodic sighs *Ref. 142, p. 41*

1146. During IMV the mechanical ventilator should be set on:
a. assist
b. assist-control
c. control
d. any of these
e. assist with PEEP *Ref. 142, p. 44*

1147. An advantage of IMV is:
a. the patient does not require sedation
b. the need for mechanical sighs is eliminated
c. multiple measurements of respiratory function are not necessary
d. assisted ventilation is not required
e. all of these *Ref. 142, p. 44*

1148. During IMV the patient's minute ventilation is governed by:

a. machine only
b. spontaneous flow only
c. manually bagging the patient
d. machine and spontaneous flow
e. none of these *Ref. 143, p. 332*

1149. Which of the following would *not* be necessary to modify a ventilator to deliver IMV?

a. one-way non-rebreathing valve
b. air-oxygen blending device
c. volume reading device
d. reservoir bag
e. humidification source *Ref. 144, p. 83*

1150. IMV can be used in:

a. infants
b. children
c. adults
d. all of these
e. a and b *Ref. 144, p. 84*

1151. IMV is useful to:

a. eliminate weaning
b. reduce the weaning time period
c. eliminate mechanical ventilation
d. eliminate controlled ventilation
e. increase the weaning time period

Ref. 143, p. 334

1152. Fighting the ventilator means:

a. the patient is not being ventilated
b. the patient is out of phase with the ventilator settings
c. the patient is assisting
d. the patient is not assisting
e. the patient does not like the ventilator

Ref. 36, p. 19

1153. When patients fight the ventilator they usually are:

a. hypoxemic
b. underventilated

c. uncomfortable because of the pressure wave form
d. suffering pain
e. all of these *Ref. 111, p. 59*

1154. Prolonged mechanical hyperventilation may lead to:
a. respiratory acidosis
b. metabolic acidosis
c. respiratory alkalosis
d. metabolic alkalosis
e. none of these *Ref. 26, p. 121*

1155. Increasing the amount of mechanical deadspace on a ventilator patient, while leaving all other settings unchanged, will:
a. decrease the patient's PCO_2
b. increase the patient's PCO_2
c. decrease the patient's PO_2
d. increase the patient's PO_2
e. increase the patient's pH *Ref. 111, p. 209*

1156. Increasing the minute ventilation of a ventilator patient will:
a. increase his pH and decrease his PO_2
b. decrease his pH and decrease his oxyhemoglobin saturation
c. increase his pH and decrease his PCO_2
d. decrease his pH and decrease his PCO_2
e. none of these *Ref. 26, p. 121*

1157. If the patient is out of phase with the lung ventilator:
a. venous return increases
b. intrathoracic pressure increases
c. intrathoracic pressure decreases
d. oxygenation increases
e. nothing happens at all *Ref. 28, p. 153*

1158. During assisted ventilation, gas flow is initiated by the patient; flow continues and recycling does not occur. The probable cause is which one of the following?

a. increased airway resistance
b. a sizeable leak in the system
c. the valve mechanism is stuck
d. decreased airway resistance
e. the flow rate is set too low *Ref. 71, p. 165*

1159. A good method of determining the adequacy of ventilation is:

a. chest excursion
b. PO_2
c. arterial blood gas studies
d. all of these
e. a and c *Ref. 26, pp. 376–77*

Using the following information, answer questions 1160 and 1161. The patient weighs 15 kg and is being ventilated with a volume-cycled ventilator. The appropriate controls are:

RR 26
assist
reading on pressure gauge 56 cm H_2O
V_T 330 ml (machine)
machine tubing compliance 4 ml/cm H_2O

1160. The actual tidal volume of the patient is:

a. 45 ml
b. 60 ml
c. 75 ml
d. 105 ml
e. 150 ml *Ref. 71, p. 163*

1161. The minute volume of the patient is:

a. 2.7 liters
b. 2730 ml
c. 7.2 liters
d. 7238 ml
e. 5 liters *Ref. 26, p. 55*

1162. The predicted tidal volume for an infant weighing 4 kg is:

a. 12 ml
b. 16 ml
c. 20 ml
d. 24 ml
e. 28 ml *Ref. 124, p. 96*

1163. Which of the following is not an indication for assisting ventilation?

a. apnea
b. hypercarbia
c. tachycardia
d. acidemia
e. hypoxemia *Ref. 55, p. 312*

1164. An indicator of the amount of arterial oxygenation is:

a. $F_{I_{O_2}}$
b. $P_{a_{O_2}}$
c. VD/VT ratio
d. FRC
e. all of these *Ref. 125, p. 225*

1165. Which of the following is not a potential complication of mechanical ventilation in infants?

a. infection
b. retrolental fibroplasia
c. bronchiolitis
d. bronchopulmonary dysplasia
e. pneumothorax *Ref. 25, p. 69*

1166. Ventilation of an intubated patient with dry, cold air results in:

a. increased viscosity of bronchial secretions
b. inhibition and repression of ciliar activity
c. bacterial infection
d. all of these
e. a and b *Ref. 109, p. 221*

1167. Which of the following drugs is used to sedate infants and children requiring mechanical ventilation?

a. morphine
b. Valium
c. diazepam
d. all of these
e. Lasix *Ref. 36, p. 18*

1168. A patient on a mechanical ventilator can be sedated by using:

a. curare
b. pancuronium bromide
c. succinylcholine chloride
d. all of these
e. a and b *Ref. 125, p. 227*

1169. Morphine and Valium should not be used in patients with:

a. air trapping
b. severe bronchospasm
c. status asthmaticus
d. bronchiolitis
e. all of these *Ref. 36, p. 19*

1170. Which of the following complications can occur when 40–50 cm H_2O pressure is used to ventilate a newborn?

a. pneumothorax
b. impaired venous return
c. tracheomalacia
d. all of these
e. a and b *Ref. 20, p. 160*

1171. The best means of determining the efficacy of the ventilator setting is to:

a. ask the patient's physician
b. monitor F_{IO_2} and expired tidal volume
c. auscultate
d. perform blood gas analysis
e. observe the rise and fall of the chest

Ref. 26, p. 376

1172. A normal V_D/V_T ratio would be:

a. 0.20
b. 0.25
c. 0.30
d. 0.40
e. all of these *Ref. 28, p. 29*

1173. Assuming the ventilator controls are not changed, what will happen to the readings on the pressure gauge as the patient's lung compliance improves?

a. they will increase
b. they will decrease
c. they will remain the same
d. none of these
e. all of these *Ref. 127, p. 126*

1174. An infant breathing 40 breaths per minute has _____ seconds for a complete respiratory cycle.

a. 0.5
b. 1.0
c. 1.5
d. 2.0
e. 2.5 *Ref. 20, p. 160*

1175. A ventilator used to function as an assistor when ventilating an infant must have a:

a. low inspiratory flow rate
b. wide range of respiratory rate control
c. rapid response time
d. large tubing compliance factor
e. volume capability up to 350 ml *Ref. 25, p. 125*

1176. When a ventilator with high inspiratory flow rates is used to ventilate infants, which of the following may occur?

a. premature delivery of volume into the system
b. generation of high system pressures
c. inadequate I/E ratios
d. alveolar hypoventilation
e. all of these *Ref. 25, p. 125*

1177. In a child undergoing mechanical ventilation via tracheostomy, the adequacy of humidity therapy is best gauged by:

a. the amount of water being used by the hour
b. the amount of water visible in the ventilator tubing
c. observing the viscosity of secretions
d. auscultation
e. chest x-ray *Ref. 107, p. 117*

1178. Which of the following conditions increases proximal pressure of a ventilator?

a. leaks
b. disconnections
c. kinking of tubes
d. power failure
e. apnea *Ref. 53, p. 201*

1179. When ventilating a newborn with a mechanical ventilator without a constant through flow, it is important to keep the humidifying device filled with water because:

a. newborns require high humidity
b. you might forget to fill it
c. the lower the water level, the greater the mechanical V_D
d. the lower the water level, the lower the mechanical V_D
e. none of these *Ref. 130*

1180. The complications of mechanical ventilation can be minimized by:

a. careful tracheobronchial toilet
b. use of low airway pressures
c. use of low oxygen concentrations
d. all of these
e. a and b *Ref. 36, p. 18*

1181. If a ventilator suddenly stops while in operation, what should you do?

a. open the patient's airway
b. call for help

c. hyperextend the patient's neck
d. manually bag the patient
e. all of these *Ref. 111, p. 63*

1182. The computation of the gas delivered to the lungs, divided by the peak airway pressure reached to deliver that volume is:
a. resistance
b. V_D/V_T ratio
c. effective dynamic compliance
d. anatomic shunt equation
e. mechanical deadspace *Ref. 28, p. 155*

1183. During mechanical ventilation, if an infant becomes cyanotic and starts to fight the ventilator, you should:
a. use sedation
b. attempt to adjust the ventilator to accomodate the infant's respiratory pattern
c. look for an obstruction
d. all of these
e. a and b *Ref. 57, p. 166*

1184. During spontaneous respiration the I/E ratio is usually:
a. 1:1
b. 1:1.5
c. 1:2
d. 1:3
e. 1:4 *Ref. 127, p. 129*

1185. Following resuscitative procedures and mechanical ventilation, the purpose of A/P and lateral chest x-rays is to:
a. confirm the position of the endotracheal tube
b. rule out pneumothorax
c. rule out other cardiopulmonary abnormalities
d. all of these
e. a and b *Ref. 33, p. 30*

1186. An example of a nonmechanical monitor is the:
a. Bennett spirometer
b. Wright respirometer
c. Ohio vortex spirometer
d. CVP catheter
e. Bourns ventilator monitor *Ref. 48, p. 96*

1187. The purpose of a Y tube in tracheal suction is to:
a. increase the efficiency of suction
b. increase the duration of negative pressure
c. reduce the duration of negative pressure
d. eliminate tracheal damage
e. none of these *Ref. 53, p. 197*

1188. What is the most sensitive index to trouble during suctioning in an infant or child?
a. hypoxia
b. atelectasis
c. tachycardia
d. bradycardia
e. respiratory rate *Ref. 110, p. 123*

1189. The effects of tracheal suction are related to the:
a. amount of negative pressure
b. duration of negative pressure
c. length of tubing
d. all of these
e. a and b *Ref. 145, p. 468*

1190. For occasional removal of secretions from an infant's pharynx during transport, you should use a:
a. DeLee mucus trap
b. Ambu pump
c. Laerdal suction unit
d. Stedman pump
e. Emerson suction *Ref. 41, p. 47*

1191. When suctioning infants from a wall-unit suction, which of the following pressures should be used?
a. 0–60 mm Hg
b. 60–100 mm Hg
c. 100–120 mm Hg

d. 120–140 mm Hg
e. 140–180 mm Hg *Ref. 146, p. 2501*

1192. When suctioning children from a portable suction unit, which of the following pressures should be used?
a. 60–100 mm Hg
b. 4–4.8 in. Hg
c. 5–10 in. Hg
d. 7–15 in. Hg
e. 120–150 mm Hg *Ref. 147, p. 617*

1193. Ideally, the diameter of a suction catheter should be ______ the inside diameter of an endotracheal or tracheostomy tube.
a. ¼
b. ⅓
c. ½
d. ⅝
e. ⅔ *Ref. 26, p. 368*

1194. In an infant, vigorous and prolonged stimulation of the posterior pharynx with a suction catheter may cause:
a. cyanosis
b. laryngospasm
c. tachycardia
d. tachypnea
e. all of these *Ref. 35, p. 204*

1195. The purpose of intratracheal instillation of saline is to:
a. prevent occlusion of the airway by secretions
b. help compensate for inadequate humidification
c. increase electrolyte balance
d. all of these
e. a and b *Ref. 35, p. 244*

1196. Following aspiration of secretions from a patient on a mechanical ventilator, the clinician should record:

a. the color, amount and odor of secretions
b. the color, amount, odor and consistency of secretions
c. catheter size, amount of subatmospheric pressure and color of sputum
d. amount of subatmospheric pressure and color of sputum
e. only the fact that the patient was suctioned

Ref. 53, p. 198

1197. A decrease in ADH will cause:

a. increased urinary output
b. decreased urinary output
c. no change in urinary output
d. polyuria
e. renal tubule dysfunction *Ref. 20, p. 162*

1198. The mechanism by which urinary output is decreased during mechanical ventilation is:

a. increased cardiac output
b. increased ADH production
c. increased renal blood flow
d. all of these
e. b and c *Ref. 26, p. 348*

1199. Fluid overload may occur during mechanical ventilation as the result of:

a. inappropriate antidiuresis
b. ultrasonic nebulization therapy
c. overzealous fluid therapy
d. all of these
e. a and c *Ref. 36, p. 19*

1200. Because respiratory rates of infants often reach 40–50 per minute, an ideal infant ventilator should have:

a. volumes as low as 2 ml
b. slow flow rates
c. fast response time
d. minimal tubing compliance
e. all of these *Ref. 4, p. 169*

Answer Key

Answers for questions 1-150

1. a	**26.** d	**51.** e	**76.** a	**101.** e	**126.** e
2. a	**27.** c	**52.** a	**77.** a	**102.** a	**127.** b
3. c	**28.** c	**53.** d	**78.** a	**103.** c	**128.** c
4. c	**29.** c	**54.** a	**79.** c	**104.** d	**129.** b
5. a	**30.** d	**55.** b	**80.** c	**105.** c	**130.** c
6. c	**31.** d	**56.** c	**81.** c	**106.** d	**131.** c
7. a	**32.** c	**57.** c	**82.** c	**107.** e	**132.** b
8. d	**33.** b	**58.** e	**83.** d	**108.** a	**133.** e
9. b	**34.** d	**59.** c	**84.** e	**109.** b	**134.** b
10. b	**35.** a	**60.** c	**85.** e	**110.** c	**135.** b
11. d	**36.** d	**61.** b	**86.** b	**111.** c	**136.** d
12. c	**37.** c	**62.** a	**87.** d	**112.** b	**137.** e
13. a	**38.** d	**63.** d	**88.** d	**113.** c	**138.** c
14. a	**39.** b	**64.** b	**89.** c	**114.** a	**139.** b
15. c	**40.** b	**65.** e	**90.** a	**115.** c	**140.** e
16. d	**41.** d	**66.** e	**91.** c	**116.** b	**141.** c
17. d	**42.** a	**67.** c	**92.** d	**117.** d	**142.** e
18. c	**43.** a	**68.** e	**93.** c	**118.** d	**143.** d
19. d	**44.** d	**69.** c	**94.** c	**119.** a	**144.** a
20. a	**45.** d	**70.** b	**95.** c	**120.** d	**145.** a
21. e	**46.** a	**71.** e	**96.** e	**121.** d	**146.** c
22. a	**47.** c	**72.** e	**97.** c	**122.** d	**147.** d
23. d	**48.** c	**73.** c	**98.** c	**123.** b	**148.** c
24. d	**49.** b	**74.** a	**99.** a	**124.** b	**149.** c
25. c	**50.** b	**75.** d	**100.** d	**125.** d	**150.** b

Answers for questions 151-300

151. a	176. c	201. h	226. e	251. d	276. b
152. c	177. b	202. i	227. d	252. a	277. d
153. b	178. c	203. o	228. f	253. e	278. e
154. c	179. c	204. p	229. a	254. d	279. e
155. c	180. c	205. n	230. b	255. a	280. d
156. e	181. b	206. f	231. d	256. b	281. a
157. b	182. a	207. h	232. c	257. e	282. c
158. c	183. a	208. d	233. e	258. c	283. b
159. c	184. b	209. e	234. b	259. b	284. b
160. d	185. e	210. l	235. c	260. d	285. d
161. a	186. b	211. j	236. e	261. a	286. b
162. d	187. d	212. k	237. b	262. a	287. b
163. b	188. d	213. i	238. e	263. c	288. a
164. a	189. b	214. a	239. d	264. b	289. a
165. e	190. d	215. b	240. c	265. e	290. b
166. a	191. e	216. c	241. c	266. b	291. a
167. c	192. f	217. g	242. c	267. b	292. a
168. c	193. c	218. c	243. e	268. e	293. d
169. c	194. g	219. g	244. e	269. d	294. e
170. e	195. a	220. d	245. d	270. b	295. d
171. c	196. b	221. e	246. a	271. c	296. d
172. a	197. j	222. f	247. e	272. c	297. c
173. e	198. l	223. a	248. e	273. b	298. c
174. a	199. k	224. b	249. c	274. c	299. a
175. c	200. m	225. c	250. c	275. b	300. b

Answers for questions 301-450

301. c	326. b	351. b	376. c	401. d	426. a
302. e	327. b	352. c	377. d	402. d	427. d
303. d	328. e	353. d	378. e	403. e	428. d
304. c	329. b	354. b	379. b	404. g	429. d
305. c	330. c	355. b	380. d	405. f	430. a
306. b	331. e	356. c	381. c	406. d	431. a
307. d	332. b	357. c	382. c	407. h	432. c
308. d	333. c	358. d	383. a	408. b	433. b
309. d	334. c	359. b	384. c	409. e	434. b
310. c	335. b	360. c	385. c	410. c	435. e
311. d	336. c	361. d	386. b	411. j	436. b
312. d	337. b	362. d	387. d	412. a	437. b
313. c	338. b	363. e	388. d	413. i	438. b
314. d	339. c	364. d	389. d	414. d	439. e
315. d	340. d	365. e	390. e	415. b	440. a
316. a	341. d	366. b	391. g	416. b	441. c
317. e	342. c	367. a	392. i	417. c	442. d
318. c	343. e	368. a	393. a	418. e	443. c
319. e	344. e	369. d	394. b	419. e	444. d
320. b	345. e	370. e	395. j	420. e	445. b
321. b	346. b	371. d	396. f	421. b	446. b
322. e	347. e	372. e	397. k	422. a	447. c
323. c	348. c	373. c	398. c	423. c	448. c
324. d	349. a	374. d	399. h	424. e	449. c
325. d	350. e	375. d	400. d	425. d	450. c

Answers for questions 451-600

451. b	**476.** a	**501.** b	**526.** a	**551.** f	**576.** l
452. d	**477.** b	**502.** c	**527.** b	**552.** i	**577.** c
453. a	**478.** d	**503.** c	**528.** d	**553.** h	**578.** a
454. c	**479.** d	**504.** b	**529.** b	**554.** c	**579.** g
455. d	**480.** b	**505.** b	**530.** c & d	**555.** g	**580.** n
456. i	**481.** d	**506.** b	**531.** b	**556.** b	**581.** b
457. h	**482.** c	**507.** c	**532.** a	**557.** j	**582.** d
458. j	**483.** d	**508.** c	**533.** b	**558.** o	**583.** a
459. k	**484.** d	**509.** d	**534.** c	**559.** t	**584.** c
460. l	**485.** e	**510.** a	**535.** d	**560.** x	**585.** d
461. m	**486.** d	**511.** b	**536.** d	**561.** p	**586.** d
462. n	**487.** d	**512.** b	**537.** c	**562.** w	**587.** c
463. b	**488.** c	**513.** b	**538.** a	**563.** m	**588.** d
464. g	**489.** d	**514.** a	**539.** c	**564.** q	**589.** c
465. a	**490.** b	**515.** e	**540.** c	**565.** d	**590.** a
466. f	**491.** d	**516.** d	**541.** c	**566.** e	**591.** e
467. c	**492.** e	**517.** c	**542.** c	**567.** r	**592.** e
468. e	**493.** d	**518.** a	**543.** a	**568.** v	**593.** e
469. o	**494.** b	**519.** e	**544.** a	**569.** i	**594.** e
470. d	**495.** e	**520.** c	**545.** b	**570.** u	**595.** c
471. c	**496.** a	**521.** b	**546.** d	**571.** k	**596.** e
472. c	**497.** b	**522.** b	**547.** d	**572.** s	**597.** a
473. d	**498.** b	**523.** d	**548.** d	**573.** j	**598.** e
474. d	**499.** c	**524.** c	**549.** e	**574.** f	**599.** e
475. d	**500.** b	**525.** a	**550.** a	**575.** h	**600.** d

Answers for questions 601-750

601. d	**626.** c	**651.** c	**676.** d	**701.** e	**726.** b
602. e	**627.** c	**652.** e	**677.** c	**702.** e	**727.** b
603. c	**628.** c	**653.** b	**678.** e	**703.** d	**728.** c
604. a	**629.** b	**654.** a	**679.** b	**704.** c	**729.** b
605. b	**630.** a	**655.** c	**680.** h	**705.** d	**730.** a
606. c	**631.** d	**656.** f	**681.** j	**706.** e	**731.** c
607. b	**632.** c	**657.** e	**682.** a	**707.** c	**732.** e
608. b	**633.** c	**658.** g	**683.** g	**708.** e	**733.** e
609. d	**634.** d	**659.** d	**684.** f	**709.** e	**734.** c
610. e	**635.** c	**660.** a	**685.** i	**710.** c	**735.** d
611. c	**636.** d	**661.** b	**686.** c	**711.** e	**736.** c
612. b	**637.** d	**662.** a	**687.** d	**712.** b	**737.** e
613. b	**638.** a	**663.** g	**688.** b	**713.** e	**738.** d
614. e	**639.** a	**664.** e	**689.** e	**714.** d	**739.** b
615. e	**640.** e	**665.** b	**690.** e	**715.** e	**740.** d
616. d	**641.** c	**666.** c	**691.** d	**716.** d	**741.** d
617. c	**642.** e	**667.** c	**692.** b	**717.** c	**742.** e
618. b	**643.** b	**668.** d	**693.** e	**718.** e	**743.** e
619. c	**644.** c	**669.** f	**694.** b	**719.** c	**744.** c
620. e	**645.** d	**670.** b	**695.** c	**720.** a	**745.** c
621. d	**646.** b	**671.** e	**696.** d	**721.** e	**746.** e
622. d	**647.** b	**672.** a	**697.** b	**722.** d	**747.** a
623. a	**648.** c	**673.** e	**698.** b	**723.** a	**748.** d
624. d	**649.** d	**674.** d	**699.** d	**724.** c	**749.** b
625. a	**650.** e	**675.** c	**700.** b	**725.** c	**750.** e

Answers for questions 751-900

751. e	**776.** d	**801.** d	**826.** b	**851.** c	**876.** e
752. d	**777.** a	**802.** b	**827.** j	**852.** d	**877.** a
753. d	**778.** c	**803.** d	**828.** f	**853.** e	**878.** d
754. e	**779.** b	**804.** a	**829.** d	**854.** e	**879.** b
755. b	**780.** e	**805.** e	**830.** c	**855.** c	**880.** d
756. e	**781.** a	**806.** a	**831.** d	**856.** b	**881.** e
757. b	**782.** d	**807.** c	**832.** d	**857.** e	**882.** d
758. d	**783.** c	**808.** a	**833.** a	**358.** e	**883.** e
759. e	**784.** d	**809.** c	**834.** e	**859.** d	**884.** b
760. e	**785.** b	**810.** a	**835.** c	**860.** b	**885.** d
761. c	**786.** a	**811.** b	**836.** c	**861.** e	**886.** c
762. b	**787.** d	**812.** c	**837.** d	**862.** d	**887.** d
763. e	**788.** d	**813.** d	**838.** a	**863.** e	**888.** b
764. d	**789.** b	**814.** d	**839.** d	**864.** c	**889.** d
765. c	**790.** a	**815.** d	**840.** e	**865.** c	**890.** d
766. a	**791.** d	**816.** b	**841.** b	**866.** e	**891.** d
767. d	**792.** e	**817.** e	**842.** a	**867.** e	**892.** b
768. a	**793.** c	**818.** e	**843.** d	**868.** b	**893.** e
769. c	**794.** b	**819.** g	**844.** c	**869.** d	**894.** c
770. e	**795.** d	**820.** d	**845.** b	**870.** b	**895.** e
771. a	**796.** e	**821.** h	**846.** c	**871.** d	**896.** c
772. a	**797.** d	**822.** e	**847.** e	**872.** b	**897.** e
773. c	**798.** b	**823.** c	**848.** e	**873.** e	**898.** d
774. e	**799.** a	**824.** a	**849.** d	**874.** d	**899.** a
775. c	**800.** c	**825.** i	**850.** d	**875.** c	**900.** e

Answers for questions 901-1050

901. e	926. b	951. d	976. a	1001. d	1026. d
902. a	927. d	952. c	977. c	1002. a	1027. c
903. d	938. e	953. e	978. a	1003. c	1028. b
904. e	929. d	954. a	979. e	1004. c	1029. c
905. c	930. c	955. b	980. c	1005. e	1030. e
906. b	931. e	956. d	981. b	1006. d	1031. a
907. d	932. d	957. d	982. d	1007. e	1032. d
908. c	933. e	958. d	983. a	1008. c	1033. a
909. e	934. e	959. c	984. e	1009. a	1034. d
910. a	935. e	960. c	985. c	1010. d	1035. b
911. c	936. d	961. d	986. d	1011. c	1036. b
912. e	937. c	962. c	987. e	1012. b	1037. b
913. e	938. b	963. c	988. d	1013. b	1038. d
914. b	939. a	964. d	989. e	1014. a	1039. c
915. c	940. c	965. d	990. d	1015. b	1040. b
916. c	941. c	966. d	991. b	1016. b	1041. d
917. c	942. e	967. d	992. c	1017. b	1042. d
918. d	943. c	968. e	993. c	1018. e	1043. e
919. d	944. e	969. f	994. c	1019. c	1044. g
920. e	945. d	970. a	995. a	1020. a	1045. b
921. c	946. d	971. b	996. b	1021. d	1046. c
922. c	947. e	972. g	997. c	1022. b	1047. a
923. a	948. c	973. c	998. a	1023. b	1048. f
924. a	949. b	974. c	999. d	1024. e	1049. c
925. b	950. e	975. c	1000. c	1025. d	1050. c

Answers for questions 1051-1200

1051. e	**1076.** d	**1101.** b	**1126.** a	**1151.** b	**1176.** e
1052. e	**1077.** e	**1102.** b	**1127.** a	**1152.** b	**1177.** c
1053. b	**1078.** e	**1103.** b	**1128.** a	**1153.** e	**1178.** c
1054. d	**1079.** d	**1104.** a	**1129.** a, b	**1154.** c	**1179.** c
1055. c	**1080.** b	**1105.** a	**1130.** b	**1155.** b	**1180.** e
1056. d	**1081.** d	**1106.** b	**1131.** a	**1156.** c	**1181.** d
1057. c	**1082.** b	**1107.** b	**1132.** a	**1157.** b	**1182.** c
1058. b	**1083.** c	**1108.** b	**1133.** e	**1158.** b	**1183.** d
1059. c	**1084.** a	**1109.** e	**1134.** d	**1159.** e	**1184.** c
1060. d	**1085.** d	**1110.** b	**1135.** a	**1160.** d	**1185.** d
1061. d	**1086.** d	**1111.** e	**1136.** a	**1161.** b	**1186.** c
1062. c	**1087.** a, b, c	**1112.** d	**1137.** b	**1162.** e	**1187.** d
1063. a	**1088.** b	**1113.** d	**1138.** a	**1163.** c	**1188.** d
1064. e	**1089.** b	**1114.** e	**1139.** c	**1164.** e	**1189.** e
1065. e	**1090.** a, b, c	**1115.** d	**1140.** b	**1165.** c	**1190.** a
1066. b	**1091.** b	**1116.** a	**1141.** c	**1166.** d	**1191.** b
1067. d	**1092.** b	**1117.** c	**1142.** d	**1167.** d	**1192.** b
1068. d	**1093.** a, b, c	**1118.** c	**1143.** c	**1168.** d	**1193.** c
1069. c	**1094.** b, c	**1119.** a	**1144.** d	**1169.** e	**1194.** b
1070. a	**1095.** b, c	**1120.** a	**1145.** d	**1170.** d	**1195.** e
1071. c	**1096.** a, b, c	**1121.** a	**1146.** c	**1171.** d	**1196.** b
1072. e	**1097.** a, b, c	**1122.** a	**1147.** e	**1172.** e	**1197.** a
1073. e	**1098.** b	**1123.** b	**1148.** d	**1173.** b	**1198.** b
1074. b	**1099.** a	**1124.** b	**1149.** c	**1174.** c	**1199.** d
1075. e	**1100.** b	**1125.** a	**1150.** d	**1175.** c	**1200.** c

REFERENCES

1. *Stedman's Medical Dictionary* (22d ed.; Baltimore: Williams & Wilkins Co., 1972).
2. Korones, S. B.: *High Risk Newborn Infants—The Basis for Intensive Nursing Care* (Saint Louis: C. V. Mosby Co., 1972).
3. American Academy of Pediatrics' Committee on Fetus and Newborn: *Hospital Care of Newborn Infants* (Evanston, Ill.: American Academy of Pediatrics, 1974).
4. Slonim, N. B., Schneider, S. N., Weng, T. R., and Fields, L. J.: *Pediatric Respiratory Therapy: An Introductory Text* (New York: Glenn Educational Medical Services, 1974).
5. Abramson, H. (ed.): *Resuscitation of the Newborn Infant* (3d ed.; Saint Louis: C. V. Mosby Co., 1973).
6. Abramson, H., and Korones, S.: Appraisal of the Newborn Infant in the Nursery, in Abramson, H. (ed.): *Resuscitation of the Newborn Infant* (3d ed.; Saint Louis: C. V. Mosby Co., 1973).
7. Marlow, D. R., and Sellew, G.: *Textbook of Pediatric Nursing* (2d ed.; Philadelphia: W. B. Saunders Co., 1965).
8. Auld, P., and Abramson, H.: Immediate Examination of the Newborn Infant in the Delivery Room, in Abramson, H. (ed.): *Resuscitation of the Newborn Infant* (3d ed.; Saint Louis: C. V. Mosby Co., 1973).
9. Wasserman, E.: Fluid and Electrolyte Therapy in the Newborn Infant, in Abramson, H. (ed.): *Resuscitation of the Newborn Infant* (2d ed.; Saint Louis: C. V. Mosby Co., 1966).
10. Hollingshead, W. H.: *Textbook of Anatomy* (2d ed.; New York: Harper & Row, 1967).
11. Guyton, A. C.: *Textbook of Medical Physiology* (4th ed.; Philadelphia: W. B. Saunders Co., 1971).
12. Slonim, N. B., and Hamilton, L. H.: *Respiratory Physiology* (2d ed.; Saint Louis: C. V. Mosby Co., 1971).

13. Kimber, D. C., Gray, C. E., Stackpole, C. E., Leavell, L. C., and Miller, M. A.: *Anatomy and Physiology* (15th ed.; New York: Macmillan Co., 1966).
14. Kuhns, L. R., and Poznanski, A. K.: Endotracheal tube position in the infant, J. Pediatr. 78:991, 1971.
15. Woodburne, R. T.: *Essentials of Human Anatomy* (New York: Oxford University Press, 1969).
16. Adriani, J., and Griggs, T. S.: An improved endotracheal tube for pediatric use, Anesthesiology 15:466, 1954.
17. Dunn, D., and Lewis, A. T.: Some important aspects of neonatal nursing related to pulmonary disease and family involvement, Pediatr. Clin. North Am. 20:481, 1973.
18. Gaskell, D. V., and Webber, B. A.: *The Brompton Hospital Guide to Chest Physiotherapy* (Oxford: Blackwell Scientific Publications, 1973).
19. West, J. B.: *Respiratory Physiology—The Essentials* (Baltimore: Williams & Wilkins Co., 1974).
20. Cox, J. M.: Prolonged pediatric ventilatory assistance and related problems, Crit. Care Med. 1:158, 1973.
21. Broennle, A. M.: New light on pediatric respiratory problems, Crit. Care Med. 2:221, 1974.
22. Bryson, M. J., Gabert, H. A., and Stenchever, M. A.: Amniotic fluid lecithin/sphingomyelin ratio as an assessment of fetal pulmonary maturity, Am. J. Obstet. Gynecol. 114:208, 1972.
23. Avery, M. E., and Fletcher, B. D.: *The Lung and Its Disorders in the Newborn Infant* (3d ed.; Philadelphia: W. B. Saunders Co., 1974).
24. Pelton, D. A., and Whalen, J. S.: Airway obstruction in infants and children, Int. Anesthesiol. Clin. Vol. 4, 1974.
25. Lough, M. D., Doershuk, C. F., and Stern, R. C. (eds.): *Pediatric Respiratory Therapy* (Chicago: Year Book Medical Publishers, 1974).
26. Egan, D. F.: *Fundamentals of Inhalation Therapy* (Saint Louis: C. V. Mosby Co., 1969).
27. Nelson, W. E., Vaughan, V. C., and McKay, R. J. (eds.): *Textbook of Pediatrics* (9th ed.; Philadelphia: W. B. Saunders Co., 1969).
28. Shapiro, B. A.: *Clinical Application of Blood Gases* (Chicago: Year Book Medical Publishers, 1973).

29. Stern, L.: The use and misuse of oxygen in newborn infants, Pediatr. Clin. North Am. 20:447, 1973.
30. Auld, P., and Abramson, H.: Immediate Examination of the Newborn Infant in the Delivery Room, in Abramson, H. (ed.): *Resuscitation of the Newborn Infant* (2d ed.; Saint Louis: C. V. Mosby Co., 1966).
31. Gutrecht, N., and Khoury, G.: Cardiopulmonary emergencies in the newborn: Diagnosis and management, Heart and Lung 2:878, 1973.
32. Vidyasagar, D.: Physiological basis and clinical implications of continuous negative chestwall pressure in hyaline membrane disease, Int. Anesthesiol. Clin. Vol. 4, 1974.
33. Harper, R. G., and Yoon, J. J.: *Handbook of Neonatology* (Chicago: Year Book Medical Publishers, 1974).
34. Stern, L.: Metabolic problems during mechanical ventilation of newborn infants, Int. Anesthesiol. Clin. 4:13, 1974.
35. Shnider, S. M., and Moya, F. (eds.): *The Anesthesiologist, Mother and Newborn* (Baltimore: Williams & Wilkins Co., 1974).
36. Mellins, R. B., *et al.*: Respiratory care in infants and children, Am. Rev. Respir. Dis. 105:4, 1972.
37. West, J. B.: *Ventilation/Blood Flow and Gas Exchange* (Philadelphia: F. A. Davis Co., 1965).
38. Comroe, J. H., Jr., Forster, R. E., II, Du Bois, A. B., Briscoe, W. A., Carlsen, E.: *The Lung: Clinical Physiology and Pulmonary Function Tests* (2d ed.; Chicago: Year Book Medical Publishers, 1962).
39. Polgar, G.: Practical pulmonary physiology, Pediatr. Clin. North Am. 20:311, 1973.
40. Brunner, L. S., Suddarth, D. S., Faries, B. B., Galligan, K. A., Lavoie, D. B., and Schwalenstocker, A. C.: *The Lippincott Manual of Nursing Practice* (Philadelphia: J. B. Lippincott Co., 1974).
41. Segal, S. (ed.): *Manual for the Transport of High-Risk Newborn Infants: Principles, Policies, Equipment, Techniques* (Vancouver: Canadian Pediatric Society, 1972).
42. *Mosby's Comprehensive Review of Nursing* (6th ed.; Saint Louis: C. V. Mosby Co., 1965).

43. Berne, R. M., and Levy, M. M.: *Cardiovascular Physiology* (2d ed.; Saint Louis: C. V. Mosby Co., 1972).
44. Hudak, C. M., Gallo, B. M., and Lohr, T. (eds.): *Critical Care Nursing* (Philadelphia: J. B. Lippincott Co., 1973).
45. Apgar, V., and James, L. S.: The First Sixty Seconds of Life, in Abramson, H. (ed.): *Resuscitation of the Newborn Infant* (3d ed.; Saint Louis: C. V. Mosby Co., 1973).
46. James, L. S., and Apgar, V.: Resuscitation Procedures in the Delivery Room, in Abramson, H. (ed.): *Resuscitation of the Newborn Infant* (2d ed.; Saint Louis: C. V. Mosby Co., 1966).
47. Ostheimer, G. W.: Delivery Room Care and Resuscitation of the Newborn, in Williams, T. J. (ed.): *Handbook of Neonatal Care* (Riverside, Calif.: Bourns, Inc., 1975).
48. Safar, P. (ed.): *Respiratory Therapy* (Philadelphia: F. A. Davis Co., 1965).
49. Collins, V. J.: *Principles of Anesthesiology* (Philadelphia: Lea & Febiger, 1966).
50. Coppel, D. L., *et al.*: The prophylactic use of a nasotracheal tube in infants under three months of age, Surgery 69:355, 1971.
51. Verhoog-Bloembergen, M. P., and Leader, G. L.: Long-term nasotracheal intubation, Int. Anesthesiol. Clin. Vol. 4, 1974.
52. Smith, P., and Daily, W.: Mechanical ventilation of newborn infants, Anesthesiology 34:128, 1971.
53. Bushnell, S. S., Bushnell, L. S., Reichle, M. J., and Skillman, J. J.: *Respiratory Intensive Care Nursing* (Boston: Little, Brown and Co., 1973).
54. Dorsch, J. A., and Dorsch, S. E.: *Understanding Anesthesia Equipment: Construction, Care and Complications* (Baltimore: Williams & Wilkins Co., 1975).
55. Gregory, G. A.: Respiratory care of newborn infants, Pediatr. Clin. North Am. 19:311, 1972.
56. Ashbaugh, D. G.: Establishment and Care of the Airway, in Petty, T. L. (ed.): *Intensive and Rehabilitative Respiratory Care—A Practical Approach to the Management of Acute and Chronic Respiratory Failure* (Philadelphia: Lea & Febiger, 1974).

57. Klaus, M., and Fanaroff, A. (eds.): *Care of the High Risk Neonate* (Philadelphia: W. B. Saunders Co., 1973).
58. Stevenson, H. (ed.): *Cardiac Arrest and Resuscitation* (Saint Louis: C. V. Mosby Co., 1974).
59. Jude, J. R., and Elam, J. O.: *Fundamentals of Cardiopulmonary Resuscitation* (Philadelphia: F. A. Davis Co., 1965).
60. Gilston, A., and Resnekov, L.: *Cardio-Respiratory Resuscitation* (Philadelphia: F. A. Davis Co., 1971).
61. Auld, P.: Resuscitation of the newborn infant, Am. J. Nurs. 74:68, 1974.
62. Standards for cardiopulmonary resuscitation and emergency cardiac care, *J.A.M.A.* 227:833, 1974.
63. Manually Operated Infant Resuscitators, *Health Devices* Pittsburgh: August, 1973.
64. *Buyer Information—Penlon Cardiff Infant Inflating Bag*, Harris-Lake, Inc., Cleveland, Ohio.
65. *Buyer Information—PMR*, Puritan Bennett Corporation, Kansas City, Missouri.
66. *Buyer Information—Ohio Hope Pediatric Resuscitator*, Ohio Medical Products, Madison, Wisconsin.
67. *Buyer Information—Resusci-Folding Bag Model RFB-II*, Laerdal Medical Corporation, Tuckahoe, New York.
68. *Buyer Information—Ohio Hope Adult Resuscitator*, Ohio Medical Products, Madison, Wisconsin.
69. *Buyer Information—Ambu with Type E-2 Valve*, Air Shields, Inc., Hatboro, Pennsylvania.
70. Cherniack, R. M., Cherniack, L., and Naimark, A.: *Respiration in Health and Disease* (2d ed.: W. B. Saunders Co., 1972).
71. Young, J. A., and Crocker, D.: *Principles and Practice of Inhalation Therapy* (Chicago: Year Book Medical Publishers, 1970).
72. Engley, F. B., and Metzgar, M. T.: Ethylene oxide sterilization: A necessity for inhalation therapy departments, Inhal. Ther. 15:10, 1970.
73. Stonehill, A. A., Krop, S., and Borick, P. M.: Buffered glutaraldehyde—a new chemical sterilizing solution, Am. J. Hosp. Pharm. 20:458, 1965.
74. Thomas, E. T.: Sterilization of Inhalation Therapy Equipment, in Dobkin, A. B. (ed.): *Ventilators and Inhalation Therapy* (Boston: Little, Brown and Co., 1972).

75. Ginsberg, F.: Ethylene oxide gas is a useful and safe hospital sterilant, Mod. Hosp. July, 1968.
76. Winters, R. W., Engel, K., and Dell, R. B.: *Acid Base Physiology in Medicine—A Self-Instruction Program* (Cleveland: The London Co., 1967).
77. Ruppel, G.: *Manual of Pulmonary Function Testing* (Saint Louis: C. V. Mosby Co., 1975).
78. Kennedy, C., and Williams, T. J.: Blood Gas Sampling Techniques, in Williams, T. J. (ed.): *Handbook of Neonatal Care* (Riverside, Calif.: Bourns, Inc., 1975).
79. Babson, S. G., and Benson, R. C.: *Management of High-Risk Pregnancy and Intensive Care of the Neonate* (2d ed.; Saint Louis: C. V. Mosby Co., 1971).
80. Fleisher, M., and Schwartz, M. K.: Use of evacuated collection tubes for routine determination of arterial blood gases and pH, Clin. Chem. 17:610, 1971.
81. Winkler, J. B., Huntington, C. G., Wells, D. E., and Befeler, B.: Influence of syringe material on arterial blood gas determinations, Chest 66:518, 1974.
82. Filley, G. F.: *Acid-Base and Blood Gas Regulation* (2d ed.: Philadelphia: Lea & Febiger, 1971).
83. Davenport, H. W.: *The ABC of Acid Base Chemistry* (4th ed.; Chicago: University of Chicago Press, 1958).
84. Ahlgren, E. W.: Environmental control of the neonate receiving intensive care, Int. Anesthesiol. Clin. 4:173, 1974.
85. Fields, L. J., Williams, T. J., and Garavaglia, M. M.: *Pharmacologic Review for Intensive Cardiopulmonary Therapy* (Sarasota: Glenn Educational Medical Services, 1975).
86. Meyers, F. H., Jawetz, E., and Goldfein, A.: *Review of Medical Pharmacology* (2d ed.; Los Altos: Lange Medical Publications, 1970).
87. Sutherland, V. C.: *A Synopsis of Pharmacology* (2d ed.; Philadelphia: W. B. Saunders Co., 1970).
88. *Buyer Information—Bronkosol*, Breon Laboratories, New York, New York.
89. Moya, F., and Lehr, D.: Drug Therapy, in Abramson, H. (ed.): *Resuscitation of the Newborn Infant* (2d ed.; Saint Louis: C. V. Mosby Co., 1966).
90. Bergersen, B. S., Krug, E. E., and Goth, A.: *Pharmacology in Nursing* (10th ed.; Saint Louis: C. V. Mosby Co., 1966).

91. Sly, M.: Drug therapy of the asthmatic child, Drug Ther., March 29, 1971.
92. James E.: Respiratory Problems, in Van Leeuwen, G. (ed.): *A Manual of Newborn Medicine* (Chicago: Year Book Medical Publishers, 1973).
93. Alfano, J.: Retrolental fibroplasia—a continuing program, Trans. Am. Acad. Ophthalmol. Otolaryngol. 74:19, 1970.
94. Coryllos, E.: Surgical Emergencies in Respiratory Difficulties of Newborn Infants, in Abramson, H. (ed.): *Resuscitation of the Newborn Infant* (2d ed.; Saint Louis: C. V. Mosby Co., 1966).
95. Levin, N.: Foreign bodies in the larynx, bronchi and esophagus, South. Med. J. 65:1099, 1972.
96. Northway, W. H., Rosan, R. C., and Porter, D. U.; Pulmonary disease following respiratory therapy of hyaline membrance disease: Bronchopulmonary dysplasia, N. Engl. J. Med. 276:357, 1967.
97. Fearon, B.: Acute obstructive laryngitis in infants and children, Hosp. Med. 5:51, 1968.
98. Crofton, J., and Douglas, A.: *Respiratory Diseases* (2d ed.; Philadelphia: F. A. Davis Co., 1971).
99. Ferguson, C. F., and Kendig, E. L.: *Disorders of the Respiratory Tract in Children, Vol. II: Pediatric Otolaryngology* (Philadelphia: W. B. Saunders Co., 1972).
100. Gould, J. B., and Williams, T. J.: Oxygen Administration, in Williams, T. J. (ed.): *Handbook of Neonatal Care* (Riverside, Calif.: Bourns, Inc., 1975).
101. Newth, C., Levison, H. and Bryan, A.: The respiratory status of children with croup, J. Pediatr. 81:1071, 1972.
102. Kattwinkel, J., Fleming, D., Cha, C. C., Fanaroff, A. A., and Klaus, M. H.: A device for administration of continuous positive airway pressure by the nasal route, Pediatrics 52:131, 1973.
103. Grenard, S.: *A Guide to the Hazards of Respiratory Therapy* (New York: Glenn Educational Medical Services, 1973).
104. *Buyer Information—Ohio Deluxe Nebulizers*, Ohio Medical Products, Madison, Wisconsin.
105. *Buyer Information—Olympic Tracheostomy Button*, Olympic Surgical Supply, Seattle, Washington.

106. Finer, S., and Williams, M. L.: Pediatric Inhalation Therapy, in Dobkin, A. B. (ed.): *Ventilators and Inhalation Therapy* (Boston: Little, Brown and Co., 1972).
107. Bendixen, H. H., Egbert, L. D., Hedley-Whyte, J., Laver, M. B., and Pontoppidan, H.: *Respiratory Care* (Saint Louis: C. V. Mosby Co., 1965).
108. Battersby, E. F., and Glover, W. J.: Management of respiratory insufficiency in infants with congenital heart disease, Int. Anesthesiol. Clin. 4:141, 1974.
109. Dick, W.: Aspects of humidification: Requirements and techniques, Int. Anesthesiol. Clin. 4:217, 1974.
110. Cox, J. M.: Techniques in Neonatal Ventilation, Int. Anesthesiol. Clin. 4:111, 1974.
111. Petty, T. L. (ed.): *Intensive and Rehabilitative Respiratory Care: A Practical Approach to the Management of Acute and Chronic Respiratory Failure* (2d ed.; Philadelphia: Lea & Febiger, 1974).
112. Hunsinger, D. L., Lisnerski, K. J., Maurizi, J. J., and Phillips, M. L.: *Respiratory Technology: A Procedure Manual* (Reston, Va.: Reston Publishing Co., 1972).
113. Ringrose, R. R., *et al.*: A hospital outbreak of *Serratia marcescens* associated with ultrasonic nebulizers, Ann. Intern. Med. 69:719, 1968.
114. McNary, R. D., and Williams, T. J.: CPAP and PEEP, in Williams, T. J. (ed.): *Handbook of Neonatal Care* (Riverside, Calif.: Bourns, Inc., 1975).
115. Gregory, G., Kitterman, J., Phibbs, R., *et al.*: Treatment of the idiopathic respiratory distress syndrome with continuous positive airway pressure, N. Engl. J. Med. 284:1333, 1971.
116. Stewart, S., Edmunds, L. H., Kirklin, J. W., and Allarde, R. R.: Spontaneous breathing with continuous positive airway pressure after open intracardiac operations in infants, J. Thorac. Cardiovasc. Surg. 65:37, 1973.
117. Ackerman, B. D., Stein, M. P., Sommer, J. S., and Schumacher, M.: Continuous positive airway pressure applied by means of a tight-fitting face mask, J. Pediatr. 85:408, 1974.
118. Rhodes, P. G., and Hall, R. T.: Continuous positive airway pressure delivered by face mask in infants with the idiopathic respiratory distress syndrome: A controlled study, Pediatrics 52:1, 1973.

119. Carden, E., and Steinback, R. B.: A new simple device for delivering CPPB to infants, Can. Anaesth. Soc. J. 21:110, 1974.
120. *Buyer Information—Fluoro-Med Newborn Infant Chamber*, The Fluorocarbon Company, Anaheim, California.
121. *Buyer Information—Infant CPAP System*, Searle Cardio-Pulmonary Systems, Inc., Emeryville, California.
122. *Buyer Information—Infant CPAP System*, Bourns Life Systems, Riverside, California.
123. Wilson, R. S., and Pontoppidan, H.: Acute respiratory failure: Diagnostic and therapeutic criteria, Crit. Care Med. 2:294, 1974.
124. Williams, T. J. (ed.): *Handbook of Neonatal Care* (Riverside, Calif.: Bourns, Inc., 1975).
125. Bendixen, H. H.: Rational ventilator modes for respiratory failure, Crit. Care Med. 2:225, 1974.
126. Reynolds, E. O.: Pressure wave form and ventilator settings for mechanical ventilation in severe hyaline membrane disease, Int. Anesthesiol. Clin. 4:259, 1974.
127. Grogono, A. W., and Byles, P. H.: Mechanical Ventilators, in Dobkin, A. B. (ed.): *Ventilators and Inhalation Therapy* (Boston: Little, Brown and Co., 1966).
128. Beck, G. J., and Grenard, S.: Mechanical Ventilators and Resuscitators, in Abramson, H. (ed.): *Resuscitation of the Newborn Infant* (3d ed.; Saint Louis: C. V. Mosby Co., 1973).
129. *Buyer Information—Baby-Bird Ventilator*, Bird Corporation, Palm Springs, California.
130. *Buyer Information—Bourns Infant Ventilator*, Bourns Life Systems, Riverside, California.
131. *Buyer Information—Amsterdam Infant Ventilator*, Isolette, Warminster, Pennsylvania.
132. Weill, H., Williams, T. B., and Burk, R. H.: Laboratory and clinical evaluation of a new volume ventilator, Chest 67:14, 1975.
133. *Buyer Information—Ohio Neonatal Ventilator*, Ohio Medical Products, Madison, Wisconsin.
134. *Buyer Information—Monaghan 225 Ventilator*, Monaghan, Littleton, Colorado.

135. *Buyer Information—Ohio 550 Ventilator*, Ohio Medical Products, Madison, Wisconsin.
136. *Buyer Information—Servo 900*, Selmedic, Greensburg, Pennsylvania.
137. *Buyer Information—Bennett MA-1 Ventilator*, Puritan Bennett Corporation, Kansas City, Missouri.
138. *Buyer Information—Gill 1 Volume Controlled Ventilator*, Chemetron Medical Products, Saint Louis, Missouri.
139. *Buyer Information—Emerson Volume Ventilator*, Cambridge, Massachusetts.
140. *Buyer Information—Engström ER-300 Ventilator*, LKB Medical, Rockville, Maryland.
141. Bancalari, E., *et al.*: Simple device for producing continuous negative pressure in infants with IRDS, Pediatrics 52:128, 1973.
142. Margand, P., and Chodoff, P.: Intermittent mandatory ventilation: An alternative weaning technic, Anesth. Analg. (Cleve.) 54:41, 1975.
143. Downs, J. B., *et al.*: Intermittent mandatory ventilation: A new approach to weaning patients from mechanical ventilators, Chest 64:332, 1973.
144. Banner, M. J., and Clarke, J. R.: IMV: Innovation in long-term ventilation, Respir. Ther. March/April, 1974.
145. Brandstater, B., and Muallem, M.: Atelectasis following tracheal suction in infants, Anesthesiology 31:468, 1969
146. Respiratory tract aspiration, Am. J. Nurs. 66:2501, 1966.
147. Williams, T. J.: Pressures and positions in suctioning, Resp. Care 20:617, 1975.

GUIDE TO REFERENCES

Acid-Base Physiology
28, 76, 82, 83

Anatomy
10, 13, 15

Cardiopulmonary Physiology—General Textbooks
11, 12, 13, 19, 38, 43

Cardiopulmonary Resuscitation
5, 58, 59, 60, 61, 62

Clinical Disease—General Textbooks
23, 70, 98, 99

Newborn Infants—General Textbooks
2, 6, 33, 35, 57, 79, 92

Pediatric Respiratory Therapy—General Textbooks
4, 25

Pharmacology
85, 86, 87, 90

Respiratory Intensive Care Nursing
2, 7, 27, 40, 53

Respiratory Therapy—General Textbooks
26, 48, 49, 71, 107